Autoimmune Liver Disease

INTERNATIONAL FALK WORKSHOP

Autoimmune Liver Disease

EDITED BY

P. Berg
Medizinische Klinik und Poliklinik
der Universität Tübingen
Abteilung Innere Medizin II
Otfried-Müller-Str. 10
D-72076 Tübingen
Germany

A.W. Lohse
I Medizinische Klinik und Poliklinik
der Universität Mainz
Langenbeckstr. 1
D-55101 Mainz
Germany

G. Tiegs
Institut für Experimentelle und
Klinische Pharmakologie und Toxikologie
der Universität Erlangen-Nürnberg
Universitätsstr. 22
D-91054 Erlangen
Germany

A. Wendel
Fakultät für Biologie
Biochemische Pharmakologie
Universität Konstanz
Universitätsstr. 10
D-78464 Konstanz
Germany

Proceedings of the International Falk Workshop held in Konstanz, Germany, January 23–24, 1997

KLUWER ACADEMIC PUBLISHERS
DORDRECHT / BOSTON / LONDON

Distributors

for the United States and Canada: Kluwer Academic Publishers, PO Box 358, Accord Station, Hingham, MA 02018-0358, USA
for all other countries: Kluwer Academic Publishers Group, Distribution Center, PO Box 322, 3300 AH Dordrecht, The Netherlands

A catalogue record for this book is available from the British Library

ISBN 0-7923-8730-9

Published in the United Kingdom by Kluwer Academic Publishers, PO Box 55, Lancaster, UK.

Kluwer Academic Publishers BV incorporates the publishing programmes of D. Reidel, Martinus Nijhoff, Dr W. Junk and MTP Press.

Typeset by Speedlith Photo Litho Ltd., Stretford, Manchester, UK
Printed and bound in Great Britain by Hartnolls Ltd., Bodmin, Cornwall.

Contents

List of Principal Contributors

B. Arnold
Deutsches Krebsforschungszentrum
Molekulare Immunologie
Im Neuenheimer Feld 280
D-69120 Heidelberg
Germany

P. Berg
Medizinische Klinik und Poliklinik der Universität Tübingen
Abteilung Innere Medizin II
Otfried-Müller-Str. 10
D-72076 Tübingen
Germany

H.-P. Dienes
Pathologisches Institut der Universität Köln
Josef-Stelzmann-Str. 9
D-50931 Köln
Germany

P.R. Galle
Abteilung Gastroenterologie
Medizinische Universitätsklinik
Klinikum der Universität Heidelberg
Bergheimer Str. 58
D-69115 Heidelberg
Germany

G. Gerken
I. Medizinische Klinik und Poliklinik der Universität Mainz
Langenbeckstr. 1
D-55131 Mainz
Germany

E.L. Krawitt
The University of Vermont
Department of Medicine
Given Medical Building
Burlington
VT 05405-0068
USA

M. Leist
Molekulare Toxikologie
Fakultät für Biologie
Universität Konstanz
Universitätsstr. 10
D-78464 Konstanz
Germany

A.W. Lohse
I. Medizinische Klinik und Poliklinik der Universität Mainz
Langenbeckstr. 1
D-55131 Mainz
Germany

I.G. McFarlane
Institute of Liver Studies
King's College Hospital
Denmark Hill
London SE5 9RS
UK

K.P. Maier
Fachbereich Gastroenterologie
Städtische Krankenanstalten
Medizinische Klinik
Postfach 608
D-73726 Esslingen
Germany

K.-H. Meyer zum Büschenfelde
I. Medizinische Klinik und Poliklinik der Universität Mainz
Langenbeckstr. 1
D-55131 Mainz
Germany

J.M. Neuberger
The Liver and Hepatobiliary Unit
The Queen Elizabeth Hospital
Edgbaston
Birmingham B15 2TH
UK

G. Tiegs
Institut für Experimentelle und Klinische
Pharmakologie und Toxikologie der
Universität Erlangen-Nürnberg
Universitätsstr. 22
D-91054 Erlangen
Germany

Preface

In recent years, there have been significant advances in our understanding of the diagnosis, pathophysiology and treatment of autoimmune liver disease. The workshop held in Konstanz, January 1997, adds an update on this subject, and a panel of experts summarize and comment on the most recent events in this field. The work of experimental immunologists is focussed on animal models, e.g. transgenic mice or by disease expression in mouse inbred strains or animals immunized with tissue extracts, hereby elucidating what kind of mechanism may govern self-tolerance or avoidance of an autoaggressive attack.

Molecular immunology has helped to identify some of the autoantigens and the epitopes on the molecules that are the target of T- and B-cell responses, and great progress has also been made in understanding the mechanisms which trigger programmed cell death, i.e. apoptosis.

On the other hand, the perspective of a clinician who has to follow and treat patients with these kind of disorders is that of an indolent onset and fluctuating course with no discernible cause, on a background of familial predisposition and female preponderance. The morphological features reveal lymphocytes attacking either periportal hepatocytes (autoimmune hepatitis) or intrahepatic biliary ductular epithelium (primary biliary cirrhosis). Often they show fibrosis of the entire biliary tree as observed in patients with primary sclerosing cholangitis. And there is still this unexplained phenomenon of why only patients with autoimmune hepatitis respond to immunosuppressive treatment and not to ursodeoxycholic acid (UDCA) while PBC patients benefit from UDCA but only occasionally from immunosuppressive therapy.

However, we still have to speculate how cells in autoimmune responses first became stimulated and whether the sensitizing agent and the autoantigen presumed to be the target of the T-cell attack are identical.

Also functional effects (or defects?) at the level of the target antigen itself may confer susceptibility or trigger autoimmune reactions and – as documented in one of the contributions in this volume – hepatocytes themselves can become capable of reacting as 'effector' cells by expressing and upregulating apoptosis-relevant ligands. These new findings may open up a new insight concerning regulation of autoimmunity, postulating that Fas ligand-mediated apoptosis may be considered as a protective mechanism or a kind of active phenomenon to protect self antigens against an autoimmune attack by being able to kill the cytotoxic autoreactive T-cells.

From genetic studies there is increasing evidence that immunological and non-immunological (background) genes exist that confer susceptibility to or protection against autoimmunity. Thus, the non-HLA susceptibility genes for autoimmunity will include genes responsible for patterns and levels of cytokine expression and also levels of expression of apoptosis-related genes and receptors for their gene products.

On the basis of those studies one could imagine that one day we might be also able to identify patients who may develop either an organ-specific autoimmune liver process or a more systemic disease, as for instance an overlap syndrome of different autoimmune liver disorders (autoimmune hepatitis/PBC, autoimmune hepatitis/PSC) or between an autoimmune liver disorder and other diseases such as thyroiditis, rheumatoid arthritis, Sjögren's syndrome and systemic sclerosis. The editors, therefore, hope that this symposium may further stimulate research in this fascinating field of autoimmune liver diseases and extend cooperation between different research groups as well as basic scientists and clinicians. That this continuous effort was not in vain is convincingly documented in the last contribution of this workshop in which it is clearly stated that the life expectancy of patients with autoimmune hepatitis – still a life-threatening condition 30 years ago – is not any more significantly different from that in an age- and sex-matched normal population provided they are carefully managed and monitored in the long term.

Finally we wish to express our great appreciation for the support received from Dr. Herbert Falk who again provided perfect organization of this meeting. We also thank Kluwer Academic Publishers for their friendly cooperation in publishing these proceedings.

Section I
Basic mechanisms of pathogenesis

1
Tolerance and autoimmunity

B. ARNOLD, A. LIMMER, J. ALFERINK, A. TAFURI and G. J. HÄMMERLING

INTRODUCTION

The processes leading from self-protection to autoimmune diseases are still poorly understood. T lymphocytes with self-destructive capacity are often found in healthy individuals indicating efficient control mechanisms.

Physical elimination of self-reactive T cells during their maturation and encounter with a self-antigen in the thymus, which results in programmed cell death (apoptosis), is one of the most important mechanisms for the establishment of self-tolerance (reviewed in Reference 1). Any antigen, whether a naturally occurring self-protein or a transgenic product, causes deletion of the corresponding thymocytes if presented by bone marrow-derived cells above a certain threshold. Besides clonal deletion, thymic tolerance can also be established by anergy (inactivation but survival) of thymocytes when the antigen is exclusively expressed on thymic epithelial cells[2–4]. In both cases, tolerance induction is based on the presence of the antigenic determinant during a stage of thymocyte maturation, rather than the result of self–non-self discrimination by the individual lymphocytes.

In addition to this central thymic tolerance, there is also a requirement for peripheral tolerance induction of those T cells that have not been silenced in the thymus, possibly because the antigen was not represented in the thymus or not present in sufficient amounts. Since soluble peripheral antigens can be taken up by major histocompatibility complex (MHC) Class II-positive cells in the thymus and induce tolerance there[5], tolerance induction in the periphery appears to be particularly important for $CD8^+$ cells, because soluble antigens usually do not enter the MHC Class I pathway. A detailed knowledge of tolerance induction in mature peripheral T cells is essential for developing strategies to silence auto-aggressive T cells in autoimmune diseases.

DISTINCT MANIFESTATIONS OF PERIPHERAL TOLERANCE

To learn whether peripheral tolerance induction occurs naturally and whether the underlying mechanisms could be useful for therapeutic strategies, transgenic mouse models were established by expressing a 'foreign' protein under tissue-specific promoter elements in non-thymic cells[6–8]. Expression of the MHC Class I K^b antigen under control of the albumin promoter, the C-reactive protein (CRP) promoter or the keratin IV promoter[9] was restricted to extrathymic tissues: hepatocytes in Alb.K^b and CRP-K^b mice, keratinocytes of the skin and tongue in 2.4kerIV.K^b mice. All these mice expressed as a second transgene a K^b-specific TCR (Des-TCR). Using TCR transgenic mice, one has the advantage of having many T cells expressing the same TCR which can be identified by anticlonotypic antibodies (Désirè-1). The Des-TCR$^+$ T cells are fully functional as they are able to reject K^b-positive skin and tumour grafts, cause graft-versus-host disease, and develop into cytotoxic T cells *in vitro*. The K^b Class I molecule was chosen as a model 'self'-antigen because Class I molecules present peptides from endogenously synthesized self-antigens and because, to the best of our knowledge, Class I molecules do not travel to other sites. The Des-TCR used here appears to see only one particular peptide[10] presented by K^b and is therefore comparable to TCR which see a well-known antigenic peptide, such as a viral peptide, in conjunction with MHC. All the mice with tissue-specific K^b expression crossed to Des-TCR mice were tolerant to K^b as indicated by their inability to reject K^b-positive skin grafts. Depending on the extrathymic tissue in which K^b was expressed, different manifestations of tolerance could be observed[11]. In the 2.4kerIV.K^b×Des-TCR mice, no phenotypic change with regard to Des-TCR and CD8 expression was found. The *in-vivo* tolerant cells responded readily to K^b in a mixed lymphocyte reaction (MLR), showing that this type of tolerance is flexible and dynamic and can be easily reversed *in vitro*. In the Alb.K^b×Des-TCR mice the Des-TCR and CD8 molecules were downregulated. These cells did not respond to antigen *in vitro*. However, Des-TCR expression could be recovered by stimulation with cross-linked anti-CD2 antibodies[11], suggesting that downregulation is mediated by a post-translational mechanism, possibly on the level of assembly.

So far, we could not distinguish between the contribution of the tissue on which the self-antigen is expressed and of the density of antigen on the individual cells to the observed manifestations of tolerance. Variation of the amount of antigen became possible by expressing K^b under the control of the CRP promoter[9] because CRP can be strongly induced with LPS or IL-6[14]. In the absence of induction, K^b expression was hardly detectable on hepatocytes of CRP.K^b mice, but was clearly visible after induction with LPS. Despite the extremely low expression of K^b before induction, the mice were tolerant as they failed to reject K^b-positive skin grafts. Apparently, almost undetectable amounts of antigen are able to induce tolerance. Thymic tolerance induction was excluded because CPR.K^b chimeric mice transplanted with a normal thymus were also tolerant in the periphery. As already observed for Alb.K^b×Des-TCR[11], this tolerance was accompanied by downregulation of the Des-TCR on about 60% of the CD8 cells. Induction of the CRP promoter with LPS led to a strong increase of K^b expression on the hepatocytes. Within 3 days after induction, all remaining CD8 cells had completely downregulated their Des-TCR[9]. LPS by itself does not lead to downregulation of the Des-TCR as controlled by Alb.K^b×Des-TCR mice which have constitutive K^b expression on hepatocytes.

These results show that non-deletional mechanisms can account for the establishment of peripheral tolerance and that peripheral T cells can reach different levels of tolerance with regard to their phenotype and their capacity for reactivation depending on the tissue and the amount of antigen expression[12].

DYNAMIC PROCESSES MAINTAINING PERIPHERAL TOLERANCE

The observed tolerance was mainly based on non-deletional mechanisms. Therefore, we asked whether continuous contact with the tolerogen was required for maintenance of the tolerant state of these T cells. Tolerant T cells from Des-TCR×2.4ker.K^b mice were transferred into the antigen-free environment of lightly irradiated BALB/C nu/nu mice. These recipients received K^b-positive skin grafts at various time points after cell transfer. Three days after transfer, most transferred cells were still tolerant because only 10% of the recipients rejected the graft. However, after 15 days, the parked cells were able to reject grafts in all recipients demonstrating that persistence of antigen is required to keep the cells in their tolerant state[13]. Thus, the *in-vivo* tolerant $CD8^+$ $clonotype^+$ T cells were not totally paralysed. This conclusion could have also been drawn from the analysis of lymphokines produced by the $CD8^+$. Des-TCR^+ T cells in tolerant Des-TCR×2.4ker.K^b mice after challenge with the K^b antigen. These cells secreted predominantly the lymphokines, IL-4 and IL-10, which are often associated with negative regulation. Whether there is a causal relationship between this lymphokine pattern and the observed tolerance is currently under investigation.

FROM AUTOREACTIVITY TO AUTOAGGRESSION

Since *in-vitro* Des-TCR+, CD8+ cells from tolerant mice became reactive towards K^b, we investigated whether tolerance could also be broken *in vivo* and whether this reversal of tolerance would lead to autoaggression. We, therefore, expressed the IL-2 and the K^b gene in syngeneic P815 (H-2^d) mastocytoma cells (P815.K^b.IL-2) and compared the growth of these tumour cells with that of only K^b-transfected P815 cells (P815.K^b) in Des-TCR×Alb.K^b-tolerant mice. The P815.K^b cells grew in these animals, whereas the IL-2-producing tumour cells (P815.K^b.IL-2) were rejected. This was due to activation of the tolerant K^b-reactive cells: when, 14 days or several weeks later, the mice received P815.K^b tumour cells, all mice rejected the tumour grafts. These studies demonstrate that simultaneous application of the tolerogen and IL-2 led to a systemic breaking of tolerance resulting in activated Des-TCR-positive cells with enhanced IL-2 receptor expression (own unpublished results). Since these mice express K^b on hepatocytes, it was of interest to see whether activation of K^b-reactive cells could result in autoaggression against the K^b-positive liver. However, no infiltration of Des-TCR+ T cells into the liver was found and no increase in alanine-aminotransferase (ALT) activity in the serum of these mice was detectable. If, however, reversal of tolerance by P815.K^b.IL-2 stimulation was followed by an infection with *Listeria monocytogenes* infiltration of Des-TCR^+ T cells in the liver could be seen. In addition, ALT levels in the serum of these animals were strongly increased in comparison with control mice only infected with *Listeria*, demonstrating acute liver damage by the K^b-reactive cells. These results have important implications for the onset of autoimmune diseases because they demonstrate that the presence of activated $CD8^+$ cells and the respective autoantigen does not necessarily result in autoaggression. Apparently, additional factors induced by inflammation and tissue damage are required.

CONCLUSIONS

The studies described here show that peripheral T cells can be rendered tolerant of antigens expressed exclusively outside the thymus. This peripheral tolerance is highly dynamic, flexible and often easily reversible. Its maintenance depends on the persistence of antigen, but it can also be reversed *in vivo* in the presence of self-antigen, provided that additional stimuli such as IL-2 are present. However, the presence of activated self-reactive $CD8^+$ T cells does not necessarily lead to autoaggression against an organ expressing the self-antigen. Inflammation and tissue damage by an unspecific immune reaction to environmental pathogens might be required in addition.

The findings on peripheral tolerance described here are not a peculiarity of transgenic mice as it is frequently observed that T cells from normal individuals (mouse and human) can be activated against a variety of self-antigens. *In vivo*, however, these self-reactive cells appear to be silent, either because the self-antigens are expressed in insufficient amounts, or because co-stimulatory signals and an appropriate inflammatory cytokine milieu are missing. Identification of the factors driving autoreactivity into autoaggression will be important for therapeutic intervention in autoimmune diseases.

References

1. Kisielow P, Boehmer H. Development and selection of T cells: facts and puzzles. Adv Immunol. 1995;58:87–209.
2. Ramsdell F, Lantz T, Fowlkes BJ. A non-deletional mechanism of thymic self tolerance. Science. 1989;46:1038–41.
3. Salaün J, Bandeira A, Khazaal I et al. Thymic epithelium tolerizes for histocompatibility antigens. Science. 1990;247:1471–5.
4. Schönrich G, Momburg F, Hämmerling GJ, Arnold B. Anergy induced by thymic medullary epithelium. Eur J Immunol. 1992;22:1687–91.
5. Zal T, Volkmann A, Stockinger B. The mechanism of tolerance induction in MHC class II restricted T cells specific for a blood borne self antigen. J Exp Med. 1994;180:2089.
6. Hämmerling GJ, Schönrich G, Momburg F et al. Non-deletional mechanisms of peripheral and central tolerance: studies with transgenic mice with tissue-specific expression of a foreign MHC class I antigen. Immunol Rev. 1991;122:47–67.
7. Miller JFAP, Morahan G. Peripheral T cell tolerance. Annu Rev Immunol. 1992;10:51–69.
8. Schönrich G, Kalinke U, Momburg F et al. Downregulation of T cell receptors on self-reactive T cells as a novel mechanism for extrathymic tolerance induction. Cell. 1991;65:293–304.
9. Ferber I, Schönrich G, Schenkel J, Mellor AL, Hämmerling GJ, Arnold B. Levels of peripheral T cell tolerance induced by different doses of tolerogen. Science. 1994;263: 674–6.
10. Tafuri A, Alferink J, Möller P, Hämmerling GJ, Arnold B. T cell awareness of paternal alloantigens during pregnancy. Science. 1995;270:630–3.
11. Schönrich G, Momburg F, Malissen M et al. Distinct mechanisms of extrathymic T cell tolerance due to differential expression of self antigen. Int Immunol 1992;4,5:581–90.

12. Arnold B, Schönrich G, Hämmerling GJ. Multiple levels of peripheral tolerance. Immunol Today. 1993;14:12–14.
13. Alferink J, Schittek B, Schönrich G, Hämmerling GJ, Arnold B. Long life span of tolerant T cells and the role of antigen in maintenance of peripheral tolerance. Int Immunol. 1995;7:331–6.
14. Ciliberto G, Arcone R, Wagner EF, Rüther U. Inducible and tissue-specific expression of human C-reactive protein in transgenic mice. EMBO J. 1987;6,13:4017–22.

2
CD95 (APO-1/Fas)-induced hepatocyte death

P.R. GALLE, S. STRAND, M. MÜLLER, H. HUG, G. OTTO, W.J. HOFMANN, P.H. KRAMMER and W. STREMMEL

INTRODUCTION

Apoptosis is a form of cell death which – in contrast to necrosis – is actively controlled. It serves as a mechanism to enable multicellular organisms to eliminate unwanted cells[1,2]. The distinct morphological features of apoptosis were first described in the early 1970s as a form of cell death occurring in liver after portal vein ligation[3]. This biological phenomenon was suggested to be of general importance in the control of tissue kinetics and termed apoptosis (Greek, meaning falling off)[4]. However, it took about two decades before the importance of active cell death became generally accepted as a mechanism to control tissue and organ cellularity in concert with its functional counterpart, mitosis.

With the inclusion of apoptosis as an active form of cell death into the cell biological concepts of growth control and tissue kinetics, cell death is separated into two distinct processes: necrosis as the result of pathological stimuli leading to uncontrolled degradation, and apoptosis as a gene-directed programme caused by physiological and pathological conditions.

Apoptosis can be mediated by a variety of different stimuli including specific receptors. Two cell-surface cytokine receptors, CD95 (Fas/APO-1) and TNFR-1 (reviewed in References 1,5,6) have been shown to trigger apoptosis by their natural ligands or specific agonist antibodies. Both death receptors are members of the tumour necrosis factor (TNF)/nerve growth factor receptor family, which also includes TNF-R2, low affinity NGFR, CD40 and CD30, among others. While family members are defined by the presence of cysteine-rich repeats in their extracellular domains, CD95 and TNFR-1 also share an intracellular region of homology, designated the 'death domain', required to signal apoptosis.

Human CD95 consists of 325 amino acids with a signal sequence at the NH_2 terminus and a membrane-spanning region in the middle of the molecule, indicating that CD95 is a type I membrane protein. In humans, the CD95 gene is located on the long arm of chromosome 10, whereas, in the mouse, the gene is on chromosome 19.

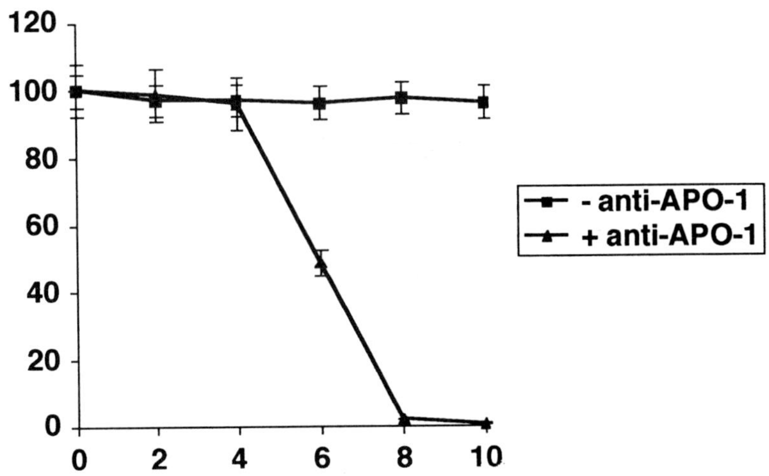

Figure 1. Stimulation of CD95 in primary human hepatocytes with the agonistic antibody anti-APO-1. After 4h of treatment with anti-APO-1, the percentage of viable cells as detected by trypan-blue staining decreases as a result of apoptotic cell death

The CD95 (APO-1/Fas) receptor/ligand system plays an important role in B and T lymphocyte development and maturation. In addition, the CD95 and the perforin system mediate T-cell cytotoxicity. CD95 is constitutively expressed in a wide range of tissues. Liver has been demonstrated to constitutively express CD95, and CD95-receptor-bearing mice rapidly die from acute hepatic failure upon CD95 stimulation[7]. We have investigated (1) the sensitivity of primary human hepatocytes to undergo CD95-mediated apoptotic cell death, (2) apoptotic cell death and expression of CD95-receptor protein and of CD95 ligand mRNA in livers from patients with acute hepatic failure of different aetiology, and (3) different regulators which are involved in CD95 receptor and ligand expression in liver cell apoptosis.

RESULTS

CD95-mediated apoptosis in human hepatocytes and in liver disease

Treatment of fresh human hepatocytes with low concentrations of agonistic antibodies against CD95 resulted in apoptosis of >95% of cultured liver cells within 4 and 7.5h (Figure 1). Immunohistology of a panel of explanted liver tissues revealed that hepatocytes in normal livers ($n=5$) and in alcoholic cirrhosis ($n=13$) expressed low constitutive levels of CD95. CD95-receptor expression was highly elevated in hepatocytes in hepatitis B virus (HBV)-related cirrhosis ($n=9$) and in acute liver failure ($n=8$). By *in-situ* hybridization, CD95 ligand (CD95L) mRNA expression was absent in normal liver but detected at high levels in livers with ongoing liver damage. In cases of HBV-related cirrhosis and acute hepatic failure,

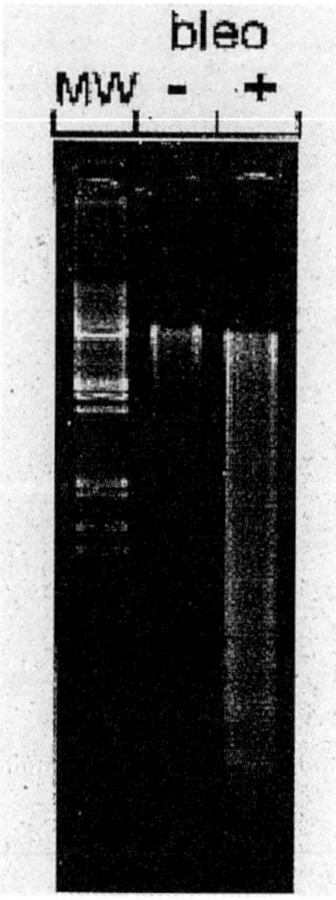

Figure 2. Bleomycin treatment of HepG2 hepatoma cells. HepG2 cells show apoptotic 'DNA-laddering' as a result of cytostatic drug treatment

CD95L expression was found primarily in areas with lymphocytic infiltration. In contrast, in patients with alcoholic liver damage, high CD95L mRNA expression was found in hepatocytes. These findings suggest that liver destruction in hepatitis B may primarily involve killing of hepatocytes by T lymphocytes using the CD95 receptor/ligand system. In alcoholic liver damage, death of hepatocytes might occur by fratricide and paracrine or autocrine mechanisms mediated by the hepatocytes themselves.

CD95-mediated apoptosis in hepatoma cells involves the tumour suppressor gene p53

For further analysis of CD95 regulation, we used an *in-vitro* model of cytostatic drug-induced apoptosis. Bleomycin treatment results in induction of apoptosis as demonstrated by 'DNA-laddering' (Figure 2) or by propidium iodide labelling (Figure 3). The response to chemotherapeutic agents was dependent on the p53 status of the hepatoma cells used. HepG2 cells (p53 wild type) were much more sensitive towards induction of apoptosis than Huh7 cells (mutant p53) or Hep3b cells (p53–/–). This was due to p53-wild-type-dependent upregulation of the CD95 receptor in hepatocytes (Figure 4) as a result of drug-induced DNA damage. In the absence of p53 or if p53 were mutated, CD95-receptor expression was unaffected but could be restored by p53-wild-type transfection. In parallel, DNA-damaging agents increased the level of CD95L mRNA. CD95 receptor blockade resulted in protection of cells treated with chemotherapeutic agents.

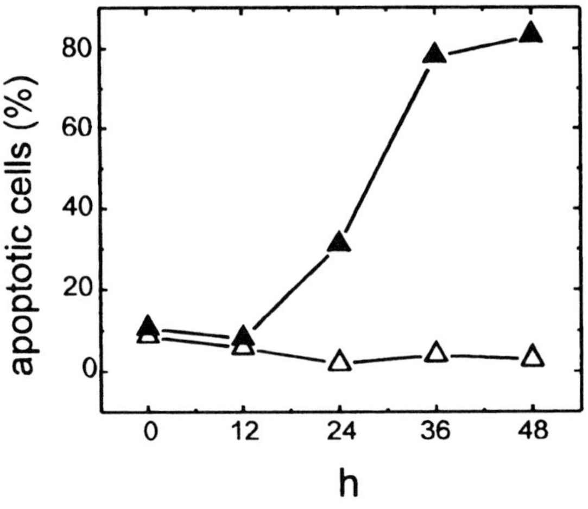

Figure 3. Quantitative analysis of apoptotic cells after treatment with bleomycin by propidium iodide staining and FACS analysis

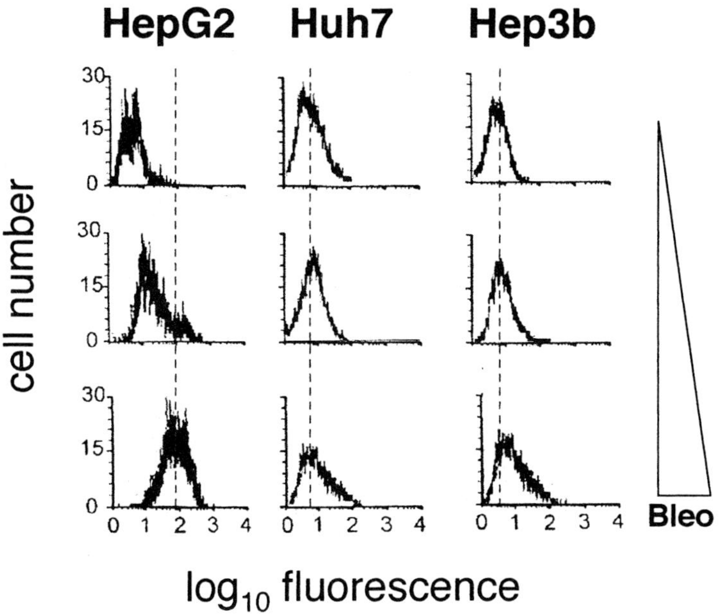

Figure 4. CD95 FACS analysis in different hepatoma cell lines in response to bleomycin treatment. Only HepG2 cells (p53 wild type) but not Huh7 cells (p53 mutant) or Hep3b cells (p53 –/–) show induction of the CD95 death receptor with increasing doses of bleomycin as demonstrated by a shift to the right

SUMMARY

In conclusion, liver cells are exquisitely sensitive towards CD95 activation and upregulated CD95 receptor and ligand levels are regularly encountered in liver disease. In viral and also in autoimmune liver disease, CD95-ligand-positive cytotoxic T lymphocytes as effector cells attack CD95-positive hepatocytes. In toxic injury, hepatocytes themselves are capable of producing CD95 ligand and might thus act both as effector and target cells in an autocrine or paracrine fashion. CD95 is directly induced by p53, a mechanism which links DNA damage as a result of toxic injury to cell elimination via apoptosis. Liver as the major detoxifying organ might use this mechanism of cell elimination to protect the organism from DNA-damaged and possibly dangerous cells.

Acknowledgements

The expert technical assistance of Young-Gyu Park, Martina Seyferth and Klaus Hexel is gratefully acknowledged. This work was supported by grants from *Forschungsförderung Heidelberg* and *Tumorzentrum Heidelberg/Mannheim* to PRG.

References

1. Steller H. Mechanisms and genes of cellular suicide. Science. 1995;267:1445–9.
2. Schulte-Hermann R, Grasl-Kraupp B, Bursch W. Apoptosis and hepatocarcinogenesis. In: Jirtle RL, Ed. Liver Regeneration and Carcinogenesis. Academic Press. 1995.
3. Kerr JFR. Shrinkage necrosis: a distinct mode of cellular death. J Pathol. 1971;105:13–20.
4. Kerr JFR, Whyllie AH, Curries AR. Apoptosis: a basic biological phenomenon with wide-ranging implications in tissue kinetics. Br J Cancer. 1972;26:239–57.
5. Nagata S, Golstein P. The Fas death factor. Science. 1995;267:1449–56.
6. Thompson CB. Apoptosis in the pathogenesis and treatment of disease. Science. 1995;267: 1456–62.
7. Ogasawara J, Watanabe Fukunaga R, Adachi M et al. Lethal effect of the anti-Fas antibody in mice. Nature. 1993;364:806–9.
8. Galle PR, Hofmann WJ, Walczak H et al. Involvement of the CD95 (APO-1/Fas) receptor and ligand in liver damage. J Exp Med. 1995;182:1223–30.
9. Müller M, Strand S, Hug H et al. Drug-induced apoptosis in hepatoma cells involves activation of p53 and is mediated by the CD95 (APO-1/Fas) receptor/ligand system. J Clin Invest. 1997; 99:403–13.
10. Strand S, Hofmann WJ, Hug H et al. Lymphocyte apoptosis induced by CD95 (APO-1/Fas) ligand expressing tumor cells – A mechanism of immune evasion? Nature Med. 1996;2(12):1361–7.

3
Receptor-mediated experimental hepatic apoptosis

M. LEIST, G. KÜNSTLE, F. GANTNER and A. WENDEL

APOPTOSIS VS. NECROSIS: DEFINITIONS AND DELIMITATIONS

Until the late 1960s, cell death was mostly regarded as a predominantly passive and barely regulated event that follows excessive disturbances of cellular homeostasis despite early pioneering studies of pathologists and developmental biologists on programmed cell death in regressing organs and during development (reviewed in Reference 1). Up to that time, mechanisms of cell death had been exclusively studied in tissues of multicellular organisms and the events following cell death on the tissue level were termed necrosis. Nowadays, cell death has become an important topic in biochemistry, cell biology, immunology and molecular biology. In these fields, the word necrosis is often used to describe a type of cell demise characterized by oedema, swelling and dysfunction of intracellular organelles, with rupture of the cell membrane and without precedent packaging and ordered fragmentation of the chromatin (in this review we follow this definition). Since the term necrosis – strictly speaking – refers to postmortem events in tissues, alternative terms such as oncosis or lytic cell death have been suggested for the description of the above mode of cell demise[1]. Although this would be historically more correct, these terms are generally little used.

A different form of cell death with a distinct morphology was first described more than 100 years ago[2–4]. This form of cell death was finally classified as an own morphological entity with distinct conceptual implications by Kerr, Wyllie and Currie, and eventually named apoptosis[5]. Its defining features are: shrinkage of the cell, detachment from neighbouring cells, preservation of the morphological structure of intracellular organelles, packaging and specific fragmentation of the chromatin, and specific cell membrane alterations indicating the readiness to be phagocytosed. Apoptosis is an inconspicuous type of cell death, allowing rapid removal of the dying cell to prevent tissue damage and inflammation that would otherwise be caused by spilt cell contents. In addition, it favours rapid reorganization of the tissue to the original structure, and avoids leakiness of epithelia such as that formed by gut brush border cells. Accordingly, patients may recover from massive (apoptotic?) hepatocyte loss during fulminant viral hepatitis without scarring[6]. In cell cultures or in pathological situations associated with an extremely high rate of synchronized apoptosis, cells cannot be taken up by phagocytosis and eventually lyse. This process of secondary lysis is often confusingly called *secondary necrosis* or *apoptotic necrosis*. However, this postmortem event does not seem to be related to necrotic/lytic/oncotic cell demise (which describes the transition from living to dead cells).

In parallel with the pathological characterization of apoptosis, developmental biologists discovered a form of 'natural', 'programmed' cell death, occurring at certain developmental stages, without severe external insult, but involving *de-novo* gene induction[7–10]. It is now clear that most developmental cell death is characterized by apoptotic morphology. The terms apoptosis and programmed cell death are therefore currently used as synonyms, although forms of programmed cell death (especially in multinucleate muscle cells) without apoptotic morphology may exist[11,12]. Notably, it is evident now that there is no absolute requirement of gene induction for programmed cell death or apoptosis to occur, since the molecular key players of death execution seem to be constitutively expressed[13]. Thus the term apoptosis has gained a conceptual aspect in addition to its original strictly morphological definition.

Recent observations suggest that apoptosis and necrosis represent only the two extremes of a continuum of different modes of cell death. It is firmly established that the same stimulus may induce either apoptosis or necrosis, depending on the metabolic situation or the intensity of the insult. This may be explained by some characteristics of the internal death program: this 'program' does not seem to be strictly linear and sequential, but rather it involves various partially independent branches, responsible for the different characteristic features of apoptotic cells (e.g. membrane changes and nuclear changes). The cell will die by pure apoptosis, if this program can be run and terminated properly and undisturbed. In contrast, necrosis or intermediate forms are observed, if the insult is so intense that only parts of the program can be executed, before unspecific events (e.g. failure of ion pumps) lead to membrane rupture. Thus, many intermediate or even completely different morphological[14] variants of cell death may exist. In experimental studies on liver cell death especially, a continuum of different modes of cell demise is often observed[15–17].

EVIDENCE FOR APOPTOSIS IN THE LIVER

Studies on the regressing or pathological liver and on isolated hepatocytes have initially contributed largely to the identification and characterization both of apoptosis and necrosis[18–23]. However, due to its inconspicuous characteristics, the widespread occurrence and relevance of apoptosis for human pathology has been generally appreciated only recently[24], in contrast to the early recognition of ischaemic or necrotic cell death.

Historical aspects

Before the term apoptosis was coined[5], the morphological appearance of this mode of cell death in the liver was called *shrinkage necrosis, Councilman bodies, chromatolysis, acidophilic bodies*, or *eosinophilic single cell necrosis*. The earliest descriptions of hepatic apoptosis date back to 1890 with the characterization of histopathology due to yellow fever[3]. Strong interest in hepatic apoptosis developed in the 1960s and the state of the art at that time is compiled in the milestone review by Kerr *et al.* in 1972[5]. The first evidence on intracellular mechanisms characteristic of apoptosis was found in 1970, when Williams described oligo-nucleosomal DNA fragmentation in embryonic liver[25]. Despite the appearance of visionary and instructive reviews[5,26], the field of apoptosis research hardly moved until the late 1980s, when new methodological approaches finally led to the explosive development seen today.

Inflammation and hepatic apoptosis

Apoptosis is a mode of cell death that generally does not favour ensuing inflammation. Accordingly, large numbers of hepatocytes may die by apoptosis without significant enzyme release or inflammation[27]. On the other hand, inflammatory mediators often induce hepatocyte apoptosis. In the liver, apoptosis and necrosis often occur simultaneously, especially with high intensity insults killing more than 20% of all hepatocytes within hours. Accordingly, apoptotic hepatocytes can be found simultaneously with typical signs of inflammation or haemorrhage.

The prototype of a general inflammatory stimulus is lipopolysaccharide (LPS). This substance has been demonstrated to induce murine hepatocyte apoptosis with concomitant necrosis upon injection of sublethal doses into mice[20]. Upon injection of lethal doses, liver damage was predominantly necrotic[28]. In addition to LPS, hepatic inflammation may also be induced by injection of D-galactosamine (GalN). This prototype liver-specific toxin acts by sensitizing the liver towards the effects of endogenous or exogenously applied LPS (reviewed in Reference 29) and has been shown to induce hepatocyte apoptosis[30–32].

In inflammatory conditions not directly induced by experimental inflammogens, there is also evidence of hepatocyte apoptosis: apoptosis is found during chronic active hepatitis[33–35] and liver allograft rejection[34,36]. In addition, TNF is induced during acute hepatitis[37,38]. TNF is a powerful inflammogen and has been shown to be a potent inducer of hepatocyte apoptosis in sensitized and non-sensitized mice[39,40].

Viral disease and apoptosis

There is ample evidence for hepatocyte apoptosis in mouse and man during viral infection[18,19,33–35,41]. Additional evidence for induction of liver damage possibly by hepatocyte apoptosis comes from the findings that viral infection strongly sensitizes the liver towards LPS toxicity[42,43], and that, under defined experimental conditions, injection of viral antigens can cause fulminant liver failure[43]. Viral infection may result in hepatocyte apoptosis by three conceptionally different mechanisms: (1) Viruses may directly induce apoptosis of cells. (2) Hepatocytes presenting viral peptides may be attacked by cytotoxic lymphocytes, that kill their target cell by apoptosis. Accordingly, lymphocytes are found in close association with apoptotic hepatocytes[44,45]. (3) Upon viral infection, hepatocytes may become sensitive towards certain apoptosis-inducing cytokines. This suggestion is based on the following lines of evidence: first, viruses may elicit the production and upregulation of proapoptotic cytokines and their receptors even within hepatocytes[35,45,46]; second, viral infection generally sensitizes cells towards TNF toxicity or TNF-induced apoptosis[47] (reviewed in References 48 and 49). Accordingly, TNF is frequently virustatic. The sensitization of cells may be explained by the transcriptional inhibition of cell-specific RNA by viruses[50]. Under the metabolic condition of transcriptional block, cells are sensitized more than 10 000 fold towards TNF-induced apoptosis[40]. In particular, it has been shown, that expression of hepatitis B virus (HBV) sensitized rat hepatocyte cell lines dose dependently towards the induction of apoptosis by tumour necrosis factor[51] and expression of HBV protein in transgenic mice sensitized hepatocytes towards TNF and IFNγ-induced apoptosis and liver damage[52].

Control of viral infection by apoptosis as opposed to necrosis would provide a considerable advantage to the body. Viral particles would not be released from dying cells but rather be digested, after phagocytosis of the membrane-enclosed apoptotic bodies. In addition, viral DNA would be destroyed by the process of oligonucleosomal DNA fragmentation that is typically found in hepatocytes killed by TNF or CD95[16,40].

Apoptosis induced by toxins and organ size regression

It was recognized[5] very early that apoptosis is not only the mode of cell death in tissue turnover and development, but that it may also be induced by stressful stimuli, by unfavourable environmental conditions, and by organ size regression[23,53–56]. Accordingly, a large number of toxins produce hepatocyte apoptosis (see below), often associated with concomitant necrosis. The significance of apoptosis has been little appreciated by many toxicologists in the past. However, in this field, the distinction between apoptosis and necrosis is not merely theoretical but has major practical implications for the interpretations of the mechanisms leading to cell death and for the design of preventive therapies.

HEPATIC APOPTOSIS ELICITED BY CYTOKINE SIGNALLING

Transforming growth factor beta (TGFβ)

TGFβ is involved in many inflammatory processes. However, it differs from classical proinflammatory cytokines in that it may also have strong anti-inflammatory[57], cytoprotective[58,59] and growth regulatory functions[60]. In the liver, it acts as a negative regulator of hepatocyte growth[55] and mediates collagen deposition by Ito cells and fibrosis[61].

TGFβ was identified as the first defined mediator, eliciting hepatocyte apoptosis[62,63]. It seems to be involved in the normal growth regulation of the liver, rather than in inflammatory or infectious hepatocyte apoptosis. Overexpression of TGFβ in transgenic mice leads to multiple tissue lesions, including hepatocyte apoptosis[64]. The acute ($\leq$16 h) toxicity of TGFβ is relatively low[17,62]. Its effects after prolonged exposure seem to depend on the metabolic situation of the liver, e.g. TGFβ-induced apoptosis is greatly enhanced *in vivo* and *in vitro* by tumour promoters, cyproterone acetate treatment or conditions of liver size regression[17,63,65]. A specific characteristic of TGFβ is the arrest of apoptotic DNA fragmentation at the level of 50 kbp fragments in rat liver[66]. This is an important example showing that oligonucleosomal DNA fragmentation is not required for the apoptotic process. In various hepatoma cell lines, TGFβ induces oligonucleosomal DNA fragmentation[67], and the related protein activin induces murine hepatic apoptosis associated with oligonucleosomal DNA fragmentation[27].

Tumour necrosis factor (TNF)

TNF is an extremely pleiotropic mediator inducing hepatic acute-phase response, hepatic regeneration and growth, stimulation of immune cells, upregulation of adhesion molecules, shock-like conditions, lipolysis, cachexia, tissue destruction and apoptotic or necrotic cell death in various cell types[68,69]. Its cellular effects are mediated by two receptors, i.e. the 55-kDa TNF-RI and the 75-kDa TNF-RII. Its signal transduction involves trimerization and consequent binding of intracellular proteins[70] to the cytoplasmic tail of the receptor. The coupling of TNF-RI by various adaptor proteins to distinct downstream signalling pathways has been characterized recently: one pathway ends with the activation of caspases, a second involves the generation of ceramide by neutral sphingomyelinase, a third involves JNK activation and a further one leads to the activation of the apoptosis-preventing transcription factor NF-κB[71,72]. It is likely that the balance of these pathways determines the cellular fate.

Studies in hepatocyte cultures

The study of TNF-induced apoptosis in isolated hepatocytes has been complicated by the fact that under standard culture conditions, TNF alone induces no or only a very low percentage of hepatocyte death[40,51,73–75]. Cell death was only observed if TNF was present in excessively high concentrations in combination with IFNγ[76,77]. This difficulty in studying TNF toxicity in hepatocyte cultures is due to the fact that TNF transmits simultaneously possible cytotoxic signals, and induces various cytoprotective mechanisms, such as the activation of NF-κB[68,69,71]. When these effects are eliminated by blocking transcription, hepatocytes become extremely sensitive towards TNF[40]. Under these conditions, 80% of all cells in culture were killed within 16 h as evidenced by enzyme leakage and loss of the ability to reduce tetrazolium salts. The typical features of cell death were chromatin condensation, budding of the cells, formation of crescent-shaped chromatin lumps and break-up of the chromatin in several apoptotic bodies. These structural changes occurred within hepatocytes which maintained their membrane integrity. In parallel to the structural changes and well before membrane lysis, the DNA started to fragment and a typical oligonucleosomal pattern of cleavage was observed. All these observations are characteristic for apoptotic cell death. Similar results, i.e. TNF-induced apoptotic cell death under the conditions of transcriptional sensitization by ActD (Figure 1), GalN or α–amanitin, were obtained in cultures of HepG2 human hepatoma cells. Examination of the signal transduction showed that neither reactive oxygen species (ROS) nor NO, nor any of various other

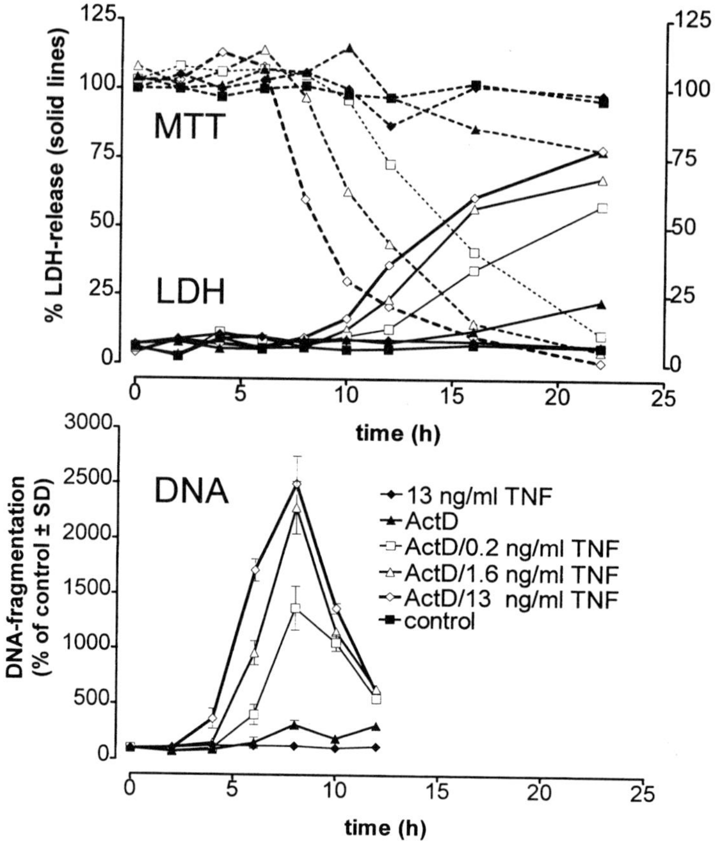

Figure 1. Time course of cell death parameters in HepG2 cells. Cells were challenged with 400 nmol/L ActD plus TNF (rhuTNFα). MTT-reduction (parameter of mitochondrial function), LDH-release (parameter for cell membrane rupture) and DNA fragmentation (parameter associated with typically apoptotic nuclear changes) were determined over a time period of 24 h. As is characteristic for apoptotic cell death, DNA fragmentation always preceded the other death parameters

well-known signal transduction cascades played a significant role as mediator of apoptotic death[40].

In-vivo *studies in mice*

TNF has been shown to be hepatotoxic in man and mice[78,79]. Mice can be dramatically sensitized by viral or bacterial infection or chemicals, such as GalN, which increased the lethality[80] and hepatotoxicity[81] of TNF in mice up to 10000-fold. The aminosugar GalN selectively depletes uridine in hepatocytes[32,82]. We showed that GalN causes a selective transcriptional inhibition in murine liver. The mechanism of sensitization towards TNF by this substance is due to the selective facilitation of hepatocyte apoptosis caused by such a transcriptional block[29]. Accordingly, selective hepatocyte apoptosis in mice was still observed when GalN was substituted by the general and non-organ-specific transcriptional inhibitor ActD[29,40]. Hepatocyte apoptosis *in vivo* developed analogously to that observed *in vitro*. Condensation, margination and fragmentation of the chromatin, associated with oligonucleosomal DNA fragmentation preceded the loss of intracellular enzymes or a drop of total glutathione levels as parameters for membrane lysis or oxidative stress, respectively[29,40]. Histological examination of the late phases of TNF-induced liver damage in mice sensitized either by GalN or ActD showed widespread necrosis, inflammation and haemorrhage. Thus, there is a sequence of events characterized by initially pure hepatocyte apoptosis that is followed by the simultaneous occurrence of apoptosis and necrosis as the liver damage proceeds to virtually complete destruction of the organ. Due to the complexity of the *in-vivo* approach, it is difficult to decide at this point (1) whether the occurrence of necrosis was due to secondary actions of TNF, possibly involving other cell types[83], (2) whether this was due to an inherent, but direct, necrosis-inducing activity of TNF, or (3) whether it was due to an incompletely terminated apoptotic program in an overstressed or energy-depleted tissue. There is some evidence for each of these possibilities. The last possibility is backed by findings that a variety of insults induce apoptosis at low intensities and cause necrosis if the intensity or duration of stress is increased[17,84–91]. In addition, we found that typically apoptotic stimuli cause necrosis of T cells if their ATP levels are reduced[92].

The large-scale induction of hepatocyte apoptosis *in vivo* and *in vitro* suggests that a very effective endogenous death program is present in hepatocytes. This can be very easily triggered under certain metabolic conditions whereas it is efficiently repressed in others. When activated appropriately, such a program may provide a means to control viral infection and tumour growth in the organ that is most heavily exposed to toxins. If activated inappropriately, it may cause rapid destruction of the organ.

Endogenous production of TNF

In the studies described above, the actions of exogenously applied TNF were examined. Similar results were obtained, when pathological situations were modelled, where TNF is released endogenously. The liver harbours the largest pool of macrophages in the body and thus it is a potent TNF-producing organ[93]. Kupffer cells within the liver may produce TNF after direct stimulation, e.g. with LPS or after interaction with activated lymphocytes in a more complicated immunological setting[94].

Accordingly, LPS injection into GalN-sensitized mice causes TNF release[95,96] and the typical sequence of selective hepatocyte apoptosis followed by widespread necrosis and enzyme release from the liver[29]. Passive immunization of mice against TNF prevented apoptosis[29] as well as transaminase release as a late sign of liver damage[29,97]. When 1000-fold higher doses of LPS were injected into non-sensitized mice, the pathological situation was different[28]. We also observed a strictly TNF-dependent liver damage associated with DNA fragmentation. However, the incidence of apoptosis was very low, liver cell types different from hepatocytes were affected, and organ damage was widespread and far from being selective for the liver. Under such excessive intensities of insult, the selective triggering of an apoptotic program may be overriden by many other processes, such as complement activation, neutrophil immigration and activation, ROS generation and many more. In addition, a possibly initiated apoptotic process may not be fully terminated to the stage of chromatin condensation due to energy failure[92].

Hepatic apoptosis was also observed in GalN-pretreated mice when T cells were polyclonally activated by stimulation of the T-cell receptor with an anti-CD3 antibody or the superantigen *Staphylococcus aureus* enterotoxin B[98]. Both stimuli strongly increased the serum TNF concentrations of mice, and passive immunization against TNF prevented this rise as well as apoptosis and other signs of liver damage. Finally, liver damage associated with hepatocyte apoptosis was induced by the polyclonal T-cell stimulator Con-A[39]. Again, the rise of serum TNF, of apoptosis, and other signs of damage were not present in mice immunized against TNF. Notably, in this model, additional sensitization of mice was not required.

CD95 (Fas/APO-1)

CD95[99,100] is the nomenclature name for a cell-surface receptor homologous to TNF-RI that was initially identified under the names APO-1[101] and Fas[102]. It shares with TNF a short intracellular domain called the 'death domain'. Upon ligand binding and trimerization of the receptor, a death-inducing signalling complex (DISC) is formed by association of several molecules to the death domain[70] and initiation of a protease cascade by one of these molecules[103,104]. The CD95 system seems to be less pleiotropic than the TNF/TNF-R system and cell death mediated by CD95 has always been described as apoptosis.

Studies in hepatocyte cultures

It was shown that injection of an agonistic monoclonal antibody against CD95 (Jo-2) into mice was lethal and associated with fulminant haemorrhagic hepatic failure[105]. Histological examination of these livers showed apoptotic hepatocytes. We were interested in whether these effects of Jo-2 were mediated directly or via other cell types and/or mediators. Therefore, we examined the action of this antibody on primary murine hepatocytes[16]. Analogous to the TNF model, a typical sequence of apoptotic events was observed with chromatin and DNA changes preceding the loss of membrane integrity and mitochondrial function. Similar results were obtained in primary human hepatocytes[45]. Notably, murine hepatocyte apoptosis induced by CD95 stimulation did not require any sensitization of the cells. HepG2 human hepatoma cells, however, required sensitization by ActD[106]. These studies suggest that hepatocytes express a second receptor that can directly trigger programmed cell death.

In-vivo *studies in mice*

RNAase protection assays showed that CD95 is highly expressed in murine livers starting in the embryonic stages, whereas RNA for the CD95L is not detectable in untreated mice[107]. There are situations when CD95L can be upregulated in the liver, e.g. after transformation to hepatocellular carcinoma[108]. Upregulation may also occur during infection/inflammation in viral or alcoholic liver disease[45] or possibly near the central vein, a region that is thought to be specialized for

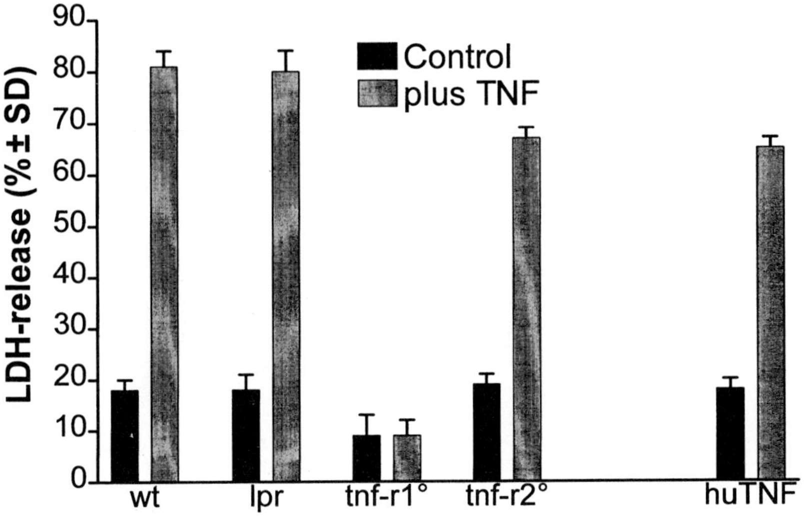

Figure 2. TNF-induced cytotoxicity in GalN-sensitized hepatocyte cultures. Hepatocytes from genotypically different mice (wt, lpr, tnf-r1°, tnf-r2°) were incubated with GalN alone (control) or with 5 mmol/L GalN plus 100 ng/ml murine TNF (plus TNF). The two columns at the right hand side indicate wt hepatocytes incubated with GalN plus human TNFα (huTNF). LDH release was determined 16 h after the start of the incubation. LDH release of unstimulated cultures was $18 \pm 2\%$

elimination of aged hepatocytes. In fact, the apoptotic index in the centrilobular region of the liver is increased[109]. Correspondingly, mice with a CD95 null mutation show liver hyperplasia due to a lack of this death pathway[110].

CD95 expressed in the liver is functional as an apoptosis-triggering receptor since the liver is the major target organ affected by systemic injection of Jo-2[105]. Subsequently, it was shown that apoptotic liver damage also occurred after injection of the CD95 ligand (CD95L) itself[111]. We examined the time course of various cell-death parameters, and whether the liver could be sensitized to CD95-triggered apoptosis by GalN. Analogous to the *in-vitro* situation, we found only a minor sensitizing effect of GalN towards CD95-mediated liver damage, but the sequence of events (chromatin changes, oligonucleosomal DNA fragmentation and subsequent enzyme release) was similar to that seen with GalN *plus* TNF[16].

Delimitation of the CD95/CD95L system and the TNF-R/TNF system

Due to the structural homology of CD95 with TNF-RI and CD95L with TNF and because of the functional redundancy, there were early suggestions that these systems would not act independently. We investigated this question by using mice or hepatocytes from mice (Figure 2) that lacked either functional CD95 (lpr) or TNF-RI (tnf-1°) or TNF-RII (tnf-R2°)[16].

(1) Hepatocytes from lpr mice reacted towards TNF just as those from wild-type (wt) mice, but were insensitive towards CD95 stimulation. Similar

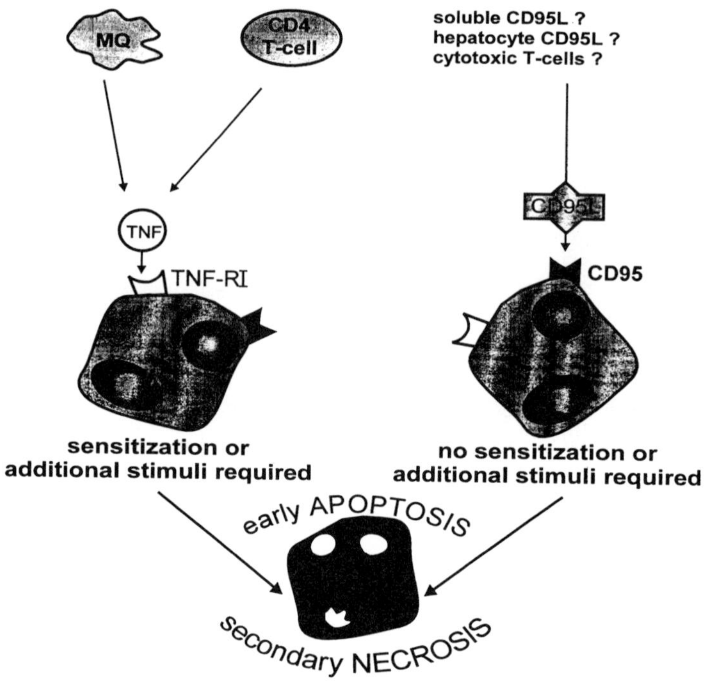

Figure 3. Two independent cytokine signals controlling hepatocyte apoptosis

results were obtained *in vivo*: lpr mice reacted normally towards exogenously injected TNF or after endogenous TNF induction due to Con-A injection, whereas they were insensitive towards CD95 stimulation.

(2) In complementary experiments, we used hepatocytes from tnf-r1° mice[16,73]. They were completely insensitive towards TNF but normally susceptible to CD95 stimulation. Similar results were obtained *in vivo*.

(3) In a third line of experiments, we tested the role of TNF-RII. Hepatocytes from tnf-2° mice were normally sensitive towards CD95 stimulation and exposure to TNF, *in vivo* or *in vitro*. It seems that TNF-RII does not play a major role in the induction of apoptosis by TNF. The transmission of the TNF death signal in hepatocytes by TNF-RI alone is further suggested by the fact that human TNF (which binds to the murine TNF-RI, but not to the murine TNF-RII) induces murine hepatocyte apoptosis *in vivo* and *in vitro*[73] (Figure 2).

These studies strongly suggest that two fully independent receptor–ligand systems control hepatocyte apoptosis (Figure 3). Additional evidence is provided by the observations that TNF apoptosis is modulated by GalN or variable ambient oxygen tensions whereas that induced by CD95 stimulation is not[16]. Furthermore, the inhibition profile upon immunological, pharmacological or genetic intervention differs between the two stimuli.

MODULATION OF HEPATIC APOPTOSIS

Modulation of hepatic apoptosis is desirable in disease control. Conversely, important mechanistic information can be derived from genetic, pharmacological and immunological intervention studies in disease models.

Pharmacological prevention of apoptosis

Since the signal transduction of CD95 and TNF-R1 has been identified only during the last two years, earlier intervention strategies could not follow a rational approach. Partial prevention of TNF-induced apoptosis in hepatocyte cultures and a reduction of liver damage *in vivo* was obtained by cAMP-raising substances[96,112]. A selective and potent reduction of TNF-induced apoptosis, but not of that induced by CD95, was obtained with fructose treatment. Liver damage due to CD95 activation was prevented by linomide, a substance possibly preventing the intracellular signalling of CD95 via the sphingomyelinase pathway[113].

The most rational pharmacological approach in the past was based on the assumption that components of the death program may require *de-novo* protein synthesis. ActD-sensitized hepatocyte cultures were indeed protected by various inhibitors of protein synthesis from TNF-induced apoptosis. Concentration-dependent protection was observed with cycloheximide, puromycin, ricin and tunicamycin[40,114]. Since these substances are chemically and mechanistically unrelated and only share their inhibitory action on (glyco)protein synthesis, *de-novo* synthesis of some (glyco)protein seems in fact to be required. Protein synthesis inhibitors alone had hardly any sensitizing effect towards TNF. Notably, these observations may be specific for TNF-challenged murine hepatocytes. When human hepatoma cells were used, they could be sensitized towards TNF by cycloheximide or ActD. Protein synthesis inhibitors did not protect from apoptosis elicited from CD95 stimulation, but rather had a sensitizing effect[115].

In 1995, the intracellular pathway leading from TNF-R stimulation to apoptosis was shown in various cell types to involve the action of caspases[116–118], a new class of proteases structurally related to the *ced-3* cell death gene of *Cenorrhabdis elegans*[119]. We and others tested whether inhibition of these proteases may be a useful pharmacological approach to stop disease processes involving hepatocyte apoptosis[106,120,121]. The result showed unanimously that both TNF- and CD95-mediated hepatic apoptosis in mice was completely prevented when caspase activities were blocked. In addition, liver damage could even be stopped after its initiation by curative application of caspase inhibitors. The *in-vitro* use of caspase inhibitors specific for different subclasses allowed a yama/caspase-3-related enzyme to be defined as a key mediator. In agreement with this, caspase-activity measurements *in vivo* showed that this enzyme was particularly activated in the liver by CD95 stimulation. Finally, it was shown that caspase inhibitors do not simply delay hepatotoxicity or shift the toxicity to another organ. Rather, a single dose was sufficient to shift 100% CD95-triggered mortality to complete long-term survival (Figure 4). Although the inhibitors used are still at an experimental stage, they suggest a completely new pharmacological approach to apoptosis-related liver disease.

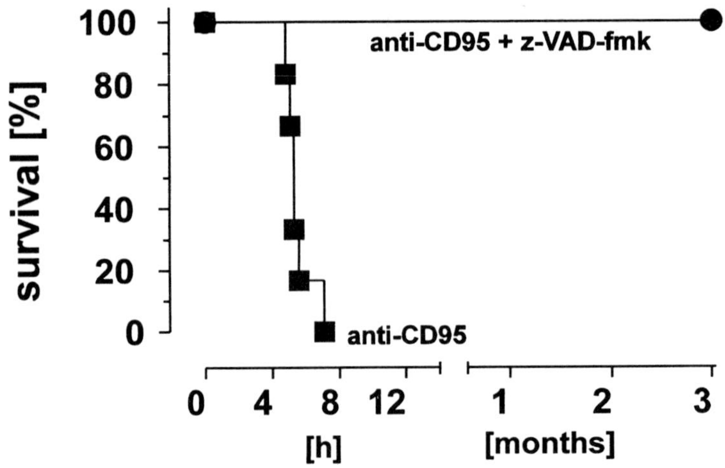

Figure 4. Prevention of lethality due to CD95 stimulation by caspase inhibition. Male BALB/c mice were intravenously injected with 10 μg anti-CD95 antibody with (●) or without (■) pretreat-ment with the caspase inhibitor (10 mg/kg) zVADfmk (intraperitoneally, 15 min before challenge). Survival was recorded over a period of 3 months

Immunological and genetic modulation of apoptosis

TNF-induced murine hepatic apoptosis *in vivo* can be inhibited by immune modulators. For example, it has been shown that injection of the NO-donor sodium nitroprusside or IL-1 completely prevented liver damage[15,29]. Conversely, inhibition of endogenous NO formation significantly enhanced TNF-dependent liver damage[15,28] so that NO seems to act as an endogenous protective substance in the liver. The effect of IL-1 is specific for TNF-induced toxicity since liver damage due to CD95 stimulation is not reduced by this cytokine[16]. Whether NO or IL-1 have an intracellular or extracellular action is not clear since the protective effect is not seen in hepatocyte cultures.

Molecules modifying the CD95 apoptosis signal inside the cell have been examined by the generation of transgenic mice. In an elegant approach, *bcl-2*, a gene controlling apoptosis upstream of the caspase cascade, was overexpressed selectively in murine livers[122]. Such transgenic mice were resistant against CD95-induced apoptosis and also lethality. This approach shows very clearly that fas-induced lethality in mice is exclusively due to stimulation of apoptosis in hepatocytes and the subsequent liver failure.

In another approach, a non-transforming mutant of SV40 T antigen was over-expressed in mice. This molecule does not transform cells but it is able to inactivate the putatively proapoptotic protein p53[123]. Hepatocytes from such mice were protected from CD95-mediated apoptosis but not from TNF. Thus, again, a variation of the two signal transduction pathways of TNF-RI and CD95 is suggested, although both have caspase activation in common. Possible involvement of p53 in CD95 killing but not in TNF-triggered apoptosis suggests that alternatives in differentiated modulation of hepatic apoptosis exist.

APOPTOSIS IN HEPATOTOXICOLOGY

Hepatotoxins may induce apoptosis[124,125] in two fundamentally different ways:

(1) *In vitro*, substances such as valinomycin[126], colchicine[127] and okadaic acid[128] directly induce cellular alterations that finally lead to apoptosis, possibly via the activation of caspases. *In vivo*, the same direct mechanisms may operate.

(2) Alternatively, toxins may lead to the stimulation of hepatocytes with pro-apoptotic cytokines, and sensitize them in parallel to the action of such mediators e.g. by weakening defence mechanisms or by inhibiting transcription.

The second, indirect mode of action has attracted little attention and will be briefly reviewed below.

Mediators derived from non-parenchymal cells and cytokines in hepatotoxicology

It seems that *in vivo* a large fraction of the most typical hepatotoxins alters the intercellular signalling (e.g. induces cytokine release or response) or acts in synergy with intercellular signals. This would imply that the explanation for their toxicity involves complex phenomena in addition to their directly damaging effect on vital structures within the ultimate target cell. The evidence for the involvement of immune mediators, non-parenchymal liver cells, and macrophage-derived products in toxicity has been compiled by Laskin and Pendino[129]. In fact, there are various studies showing that modulation of macrophage function or neutralization of immune mediators alters xenobiotic-induced toxicity. One of the most prominent mediators is the proapoptotic cytokine TNF.

Toxin-induced apoptosis

Evidence is accumulating that many xenobiotics cause apoptosis or symptoms of hepatocyte apoptosis in rodents[124,125,130–136]. This suggests that the default mode of demise for hepatocytes is apoptosis, as for many other cell types. Intoxication so severe that the apoptotic program could not be continued to the end would accordingly induce necrosis.

TNF as a mediator of toxin-induced apoptosis

If a single toxin were to release TNF and simultaneously sensitize cells towards the apoptotic actions of this cytokine, then TNF-induced hepatocyte apoptosis should contribute significantly to overall toxicity. For some toxins, such a scenario has been demonstrated. For example, the toxicity of CCl_4, the prototype of a directly acting hepatotoxin, is inhibited by scavenging of TNF with recombinant soluble TNF-receptor constructs[137].

In a parallel study, we examined the role of TNF and hepatocyte apoptosis during the poisoning of mice with α-amanitin or with ActD, respectively[138]. Indeed, the two toxins behaved similarly. At low doses, they induced hepatocyte apoptosis *in vivo* and *in vitro* highly synergistically with TNF. At high doses, they induced liver damage alone; this was associated with the occurrence of apoptotic hepatocytes and oligonucleosomal DNA fragmentation. This toxicity was inhibited by passive immunization of mice against TNF or by IL-1 pretreatment. To further confirm the necessity of TNF for hepatotoxicity, we used tnf-r1° mice which were resistant and tnf-r2° mice which were highly sensitive to α-amanitin. Thus, different lines of evidence suggest that hepatotoxicity of ActD or α-amanitin, a prototype 'direct-acting' hepatotoxin, involves the actions of TNF, in particular the induction of apoptosis in hepatocytes.

Acknowledgements

We are grateful to Ms C. Hoffmann for help in the preparation of the manuscript and to Professor P. Nicotera for stimulating discussion.

References

1. Majno G, Joris I. Apoptosis, oncosis, and necrosis. An overview of cell death. Am J Pathol. 1995; 146:3–15.
2. Flemming W. Über die Bildung von Richtungsfiguren in Säugetiereiern beim Untergang Graaf'scher Follikel. Arch Anat Physiol (Anat Abt). 1885;221–44 (*plus* Taf. X and XI).
3. Councilman WT. Report on the etiology and prevention of yellow fever. In: Sternberg GM, ed. United States Marine Hospital Service, Treasury Department, Document No. 1328 (Public health Bulletin 2). Washington: Government Printing Office. 1890;151–9.
4. Nissen F. Über das Verhalten der Kerne in den Milchdrüsenzellen bei der Absonderung. Arch Mikroskop Anat. 1886;26:337–42.
5. Kerr JF, Wyllie AH, Currie AR. Apoptosis: A basic biological phenomenon with wide ranging implications in tissue kinetics. Br J Cancer. 1972;26:239–47.
6. Karvountzis GG, Redeker AG, Peters RL. Long-term follow-up studies of patients surviving fulminant viral hepatitis. Gastroenterology. 1974;67:870–7.
7. Glücksmann A. Cell death in normal vertebrate ontogeny. Biol Rev Camb Philos Soc. 1951; 26:59–86.
8. Schwartz LM, Osborne BA. Programmed cell death, apoptosis and killer genes. Immunol Today. 1993;14:582–90.
9. Saunders JW. Death in embryonic systems. Science. 1966;154:604–12.
10. Lockshin RA, Beaulaton J. Programmed cell death. Life Sci. 1974;15:1549–65.
11. Schwartz LM, Smith SW, Jones MEE, Osborne BA. Do all programmed cell deaths occur via apoptosis? Proc Natl Acad Sci USA. 1993;90:980–4.
12. Lockshin RA, Williams CM. Programmed cell death. I. Cytology of degeneration in the intersegmental muscles of the pernyi silkmoth. J Inst Physiol. 1965;11:123–33.
13. Weil M, Jacobson MD, Coles HSR et al. Constitutive expression of the machinery for programmed cell death. J Cell Biol. 1996;133:1053–9.
14. Leist M, Wendel A. A novel mechanism of murine hepatocyte death inducible by concanavalin A. J Hepatol. 1996;25:948–59.
15. Bohlinger I, Leist M, Barsig J, Uhlig S, Tiegs G, Wendel A. Interleukin-1 and nitric oxide protect against tumor necrosis-factor alpha-induced liver injury through distinct pathways. Hepatology. 1995;22:1829–37.
16. Leist M, Gantner F, Künstle G et al. The 55 kD tumor necrosis factor receptor and CD95 independently signal murine hepatocyte apoptosis and subsequent liver failure. Mol Med. 1996; 2:109–24.
17. Oberhammer F, Nagy P, Tiefenbacher R et al. The antiandrogen cyproterone acetate induces synthesis of transforming factor beta-1 in the parenchymal cells of the liver accompanied by an

enhanced sensitivity to undergo apoptosis and necrosis without inflammation. Hepatology. 1996; 23:329–37.

18. Svoboda D, Nielson A, Werder A, Higginson J. An electron microscopic study of viral hepatitis in mice. Am J Pathol. 1962;41:205–24.
19. Klion FM, Schaffner F. The ultrastructure of acidophilic bodies. Am J Pathol. 1966;48:755–65.
20. Levy E, Slusser RJ, Ruebner BH. Hepatic changes produced by a single dose of endotoxin in the mouse. Am J Pathol. 1968;52:477–502.
21. Kehrer JP, Jones DP, Lemasters JJ, Farber JL, Jaeschke H. Contemporary issues in toxicology. Mechanisms of hypoxic cell injury. Toxicol Appl Pharmacol. 190;106:165–78.
22. Orrenius S, McConkey DJ, Bellomo G, Nicotera P. Role of Ca^{2+} in toxic cell killing. Trends Pharmacol Sci. 1989;10:281–5.
23. Kerr JFR. Shrinkage necrosis: a distinct mode of cellular death. J Pathol. 1971;105:13–22.
24. Que FG, Gores FJ. Cell death by apoptosis: basic concepts and disease relevance for the gastroenterologist. Gastroenterology. 1996;110:1238–43.
25. Williamson R. Properties of rapidly labelled deoxyribonucleic acid fragments isolated from the cytoplasm of primary cultures of embryonic mouse liver cells. J Mol Biol. 1970;51:157–68.
26. Wyllie AH, Kerr JF, Currie AR. Cell death: the significance of apoptosis. Int Rev Cytol. 1980; 68:251–306.
27. Hully JR, Chang L, Schwall RH, Widmer HR, Terrell TG, Gillett NA. Induction of apoptosis in the murine liver with recombinant human activin A. Hepatology. 1994;20:854–61.
28. Bohlinger I, Leist M, Gantner F, Angermüller S, Tiegs G, Wendel A. DNA-fragmentation in mouse organs during endotoxic shock. Am J Pathol. 1996;149:1381–93.
29. Leist M, Gantner F, Bohlinger I, Tiegs G, Germann PG, Wendel A. Tumor necrosis factor-induced hepatocyte apoptosis precedes liver failure in experimental murine shock models. Am J Pathol. 1995;146:1220–34.
30. Reutter W, Bauer CH, Lesch R. On the mechanism of action of galactosamine: different response to d-galactosamine of rat liver during development. Naturwissenschaften. 1970;57:674–5.
31. Reutter W, Lesch R, Keppler D, Decker K. Galactosamine-hepatitis. Naturwissenschaften. 1968; 55:497.
32. Keppler D, Lesch R, Reutter W, Decker K. Experimental hepatitis induced by D-galactosamine. Exp Mol Pathol. 1968;9:279–90.
33. Kerr JFR, Searle J, Halliday WJ et al. The nature of piecemeal necrosis in chronic active hepatitis. Lancet. 1979;2:827–8.
34. Searle J, Kerr JFR, Bishop CJ. Necrosis and apoptosis: distinct modes of cell death with fundamentally different significance. Pathol Ann. 1982;17:229–59.
35. Hiramatsu N, Hayashi N, Katayama K et al. Immunohistochemical detection of fas antigen in liver tissue of patients with chronic hepatitis C. Hepatology. 1994;19:1354–9.
36. Krams SM, Egawa H, Quinn MB, Villnueva JC, Garcia-Kennedy R, Martinez OM. Apoptosis as a mechanism of cell death in liver allograft rejection. Transplantation. 1995;59:621–5.
37. Torre D, Zeroli C, Giola M et al. Serum levels of interleukin-1 alpha, interleukin-1 beta, interleukin-6, and tumor necrosis factor in patients with acute viral hepatitis. Clin Infect Dis. 1994;18: 194–8.
38. Ding-feng Z, Hong R, Xiao-ping J, Ya-su Z. Serum tumor necrosis factor (TNF) in the pathogenesis of clinical hepatic failure of HCV and/or HBV infection. Chinese Med J. 1993;106:335–8.
39. Gantner F, Leist M, Lohse AW, Germann PG, Tiegs G. Concanavalin A-induced T cell-mediated hepatic injury in mice: the role of tumor necrosis factor. Hepatology. 1995;21:190–8.
40. Leist M, Gantner F, Bohlinger I, German PG, Tiegs G, Wendel A. Murine hepatocyte apoptosis induced in vitro and in vivo by TNF-alpha requires transcriptional arrest. J Immunol. 1994;153: 1778–87.
41. Child P, Ruiz LA. Acidophilic bodies. Their chemical and physical nature in patients with Bolivian hemorrhagic fever. Arch Pathol. 1968;85:45– 50.
42. Gut J, Schmitt S, Bingen A, Anton M, Kirn A. Probable role of endogenous endotoxins in hepatocytolysis during murine hepatitis caused by frog virus 3. J Infect Dis. 1984;149:621–9.
43. Mori W, Aoki N, Shiga J. Acute hepatic cell necrosis experimentally produced by viral agents in rabbits. Am J Pathol. 1981;103:31–8.
44. Bathal PS, Powell LW, Mackay IR. Apoptosis in autoimmune chronic active hepatitis (CAH). Hepatology. 1982;2:154–5.
45. Galle PR, Hofmann WJ, Walczak H et al. Involvement of the CD95 (APO-1/Fas) receptor and ligand in liver damage. J Exp Med. 1995;182:1223–30.

46. González-Amaro R, Garcia-Monzón C, Garcia-Buey L et al. Induction of tumor necrosis factor alpha by human hepatocytes in chronic viral hepatitis. J Exp Med. 1994;179:841–8.
47. Ohno K, Nakano T, Matsumoto Y et al. Apoptosis induced by tumor necrosis factor in cells chronically infected with feline immunodeficiency virus. J Virol. 1993;67:2429–33.
48. Wong GHW, Kamb A, Goeddel DV. Antiviral properties of TNF. In: Beutler B, ed. Tumor Necrosis Factors. The Molecules and their Emerging Role in Medicine. New York: Raven Press Ltd.; 1992: 371–82.
49. Rubin BY. TNF and viruses: multiple interrelationships. In: Aggarwal BB, Vilcek J, eds. Tumor Necrosis Factors. Structure, Function and Mechanisms of Action. New York: Marcel Dekker, Inc.; 1992:331–40.
50. Huang AS, Wagner RR. Inhibition of cellular RNA synthesis by non-replicating vesicular stomatitis virus. Proc Natl Acad Sci USA. 1965;54:1579–85.
51. Guilhot S, Miller T, Cornman G, Isom HC. Apoptosis induced by tumor necrosis factor-alpha in rat hepatocyte cell lines expressing hepatitis B virus. Am J Pathol. 1996;148:801–14.
52. Gilles PN, Guerrette DL, Ulevitch RJ, Schreiber RD, Chisari FV. HBsAg retention sensitizes the hepatocyte to injury by physiological concentrations of interferon-gamma. Hepatology. 1992;16: 655–63.
53. Ledda-Columbano GM, Shinozuka H, Katyal SL, Columbano A. Cell proliferation, cell death and hepatocarcinogenesis. Cell Death Differ. 1996;3:17–22.
54. Columbano A, Ledda-Columbano GM, Coni PP et al. Occurrence of cell death (apoptosis) during the involution of liver hyperplasia. Lab Invest. 1985;52:670–5.
55. Bursch W, Oberhammer F, Schulte-Hermann R. Cell death by apoptosis and its protective role against disease. Trends Pharmacol Sci. 1992;13:245–51.
56. Grasl Kraupp B, Bursch W, Ruttkay Nedecky B, Wagner A, Lauer B, Schulte Hermann R. Food restriction eliminates preneoplastic cells through apoptosis and antagonizes carcinogenesis in rat liver. Proc Natl Acad Sci USA. 1994;91:9995–9.
57. Randow F, Syrbe U, Meisel C et al. Mechanism of endotoxin densensitization: Involvement of interleukin 10 and transforming growth factor beta. J Exp Med. 1995;181:1887–92.
58. Prehn JHM, Bindokas VP, Marcuccilli CJ, Krajewski S, Reed JC, Miller RJ. Regulation of neuronal Bcl-2 protein expression and calcium homeostasis by transforming growth factor type beta confers wide-ranging protection on rat hippocampal neurons. Proc Natl Acad Sci USA. 1994;91: 12599–603.
59. Merrill JE, Zimmerman RP. Natural and induced cytotoxicity of oligodendrocytes by microglia is inhibitable by TGFbeta. GLIA. 1991;4:327–31.
60. Bedossa P, Peltier E, Terris B, Franco D, Poynard T. Transforming growth factor-beta 1 (TGF-beta1) and TGF-beta1 receptors in normal, cirrhotic, and neoplastic human livers. Hepatology. 1995;21:7560–6.
61. Weiner FR, Giambrone M, Czaja MJ et al. Ito-cell gene expression and collagen regulation. Hepatology. 1990;11:111–20.
62. Oberhammer FA, Pavelka M, Sharma S et al. Induction of apoptosis in cultured hepatocytes and in regressing liver by transforming growth factor $\beta 1$. Proc Natl Acad Sci USA. 1992;89:5408–12.
63. Oberhammer F, Bursch W, Tiefenbacher R et al. Apoptosis is induced by transforming growth factor-beta1 within 5 hours in regressing liver without significant fragmentation of the DNA. Hepatology. 1993;18:1238–46.
64. Sanderson M, Factor V, Nagy P et al. Hepatic expression of mature transforming growth factor beta1 in transgenic mice results in multiple tissue lesions. Proc Natl Acad Sci USA. 1995;92: 2572–6.
65. Oberhammer FA, Qin H. Effect of three tumor promoters on the stability of hepatocyte cultures and apoptosis after transforming growth factor-beta1. Carcinogenesis. 1995;16:1363–71.
66. Oberhammer F, Wilson JW, Dive C et al. Apoptotic death in epithelial cells: cleavage of DNA to 300 and/or 50 kb fragments prior to or in the absence of internucleosomal fragmentation. EMBO J. 1993;12:3679–84.
67. Lin J-K, Chou C-K. In vitro apoptosis in the human hepatoma cell line induced by transforming growth factor beta-1. Cancer Res. 1992;52:385–8.
68. Beutler B, ed. Tumor Necrosis Factors. The Molecules and their Emerging Role in Medicine. New York: Raven Press; 1992.
69. Aggarwal BB, Vilcek J, eds. Tumor Necrosis Factors. Structure, Function and Mechanisms of Action. New York: Marcel Dekker, Inc.; 1992.

70. Peter ME, Kischkel FC, Hellbardt S, Chinnaiyan AM, Krammer PH, Dixit VM. CD95(APO-1/Fas)-associating signalling proteins. Cell Death Diff. 1996;3:161–70.
71. Zheng-gang L, Hsu H, Goeddel DV, Karin M. Dissection of TNF receptor 1 effector functions: JNK activation is not linked to apoptosis while NF-kB activation prevents cell death. Cell. 1996; 87:565–76.
72. Adam-Klages S, Adam D, Wiegmann K et al. FAN, a novel WD-repeat protein, couples the p55 TNF-receptor to neutral sphingomyelinase. Cell. 1996;86:937–47.
73. Leist M, Gantner F, Jilg S, Wendel A. Activation of the 55 kDa TNF-receptor is necessary and sufficient for TNF-induced liver failure, hepatocyte apoptosis and nitrite release. J Immunol. 1995;154:1307–16.
74. Stadler J, Bentz BG, Harbrecht BG et al. Tumor necrosis factor alpha inhibits hepatocyte mitochondrial respiration. Ann Surg. 1992;216:539–46.
75. Shinagawa T, Yoshioka K, Kakumu S et al. Apoptosis in cultured rat hepatocytes: The effect of tumour necrosis factor alpha and interferon gamma. J Pathol. 1991;165:247–53.
76. Adamson GM, Billings RE. Cytokine toxicity and induction of NO synthase activity in cultured mouse hepatocytes. Toxicol Appl Pharmacol. 1993;119:100–7.
77. Adamson GM, Billings RE. Tumor necrosis factor induced oxidative stress in isolated mouse hepatocytes. Arch Biochem Biophys. 1992;294:223–9.
78. Jones AL, Selby P. Tumor necrosis factor: clinical relevance. Cancer Surv. 1989;8:817–36.
79. Talmadge JE, Bowesox O, Tribble H, Lee SH, Shepard M, Liggitt D. Toxicity of tumor necrosis factor is synergistic with gamma-interferon and can be reduced with cyclo-oxygenase inhibitors. Am J Pathol. 1987;128:410–25.
80. Lehmann V, Freudenberg MA, Galanos C. Lethal toxicity of lipopolysaccharide and tumor necrosis factor in normal and d-galactosamine-treated mice. J Exp Med. 1987;165:657–63.
81. Tiegs G, Wolter M, Wendel A. Tumor necrosis factor is a terminal mediator in galactosamine/endotoxin-induced hepatitis in mice. Biochem Pharmacol. 1989;38:627–31.
82. Decker K, Keppler D. Galactosamine hepatitis: key role of the nucleotide deficiency period in the pathogenesis of cell injury and cell death. Rev Physiol Biochem Pharmacol. 1974;71:77–100.
83. Sauer A, Hartung T, Aigner J, Wendel A. Endotoxin-inducible granulocyte-mediated hepatotoxicity requires adhesion and serine protease release. J Leukocyte Biol. 1996;60:633–43.
84. Dypbukt JM, Ankarcrona M, Burkitt M et al. Different prooxidant levels stimulate growth, trigger apoptosis, or produce necrosis of insulin-secreting RINm5F cells. J Biol Chem. 1994;269: 30533–60.
85. Ankarcrona M, Dypbukt JM, Bonfoco E et al. Glutamate-induced neuronal death: a succession of necrosis or apoptosis depending on mitochondrial function. Neuron. 1995;15:961–73.
86. Bonfoco E, Krainc D, Ankarcrona M, Nicotera P, Lipton SA. Apoptosis and necrosis: two distinct events induced respectively by mild and intense insults with NMDA or nitric oxide/superoxide in cortical cell cultures. Proc Natl Acad Sci USA. 1995;92:72162–6.
87. Shimizu S, Eguchi Y, Kamiike W et al. Induction of apoptosis as well as necrosis by hypoxia and predominant prevention of apoptosis by Bcl-2 and Bcl-XL. Cancer Res. 1996;56:2161–6.
88. Hartley A, Stone JM, Heron C, Cooper JM, Schapira AHV. Complex I inhibitors induce dose-dependent apoptosis in PC12 cells: relevance to Parkinson's disease. J Neurochem. 1994;63: 1987–90.
89. Lennon SV, Martin SJ, Cotter TG. Dose-dependent induction of apoptosis in human tumor cell lines by widely diverging stimuli. Cell Prolif. 1991;24:203–14.
90. Jensen JC, Pogrebniak HW, Pass HI et al. Role of tumor necrosis factor in oxygen toxicity. J Appl Physiol. 1992;5:1902–7.
91. Corcoran GB, Ray SD. Contemporary issues in toxicology. The role of the nucleus and other compartments in toxic cell death produced by alkylating hepatotoxicants. Toxicol Appl Pharmacol. 1992;113:167–83.
92. Leist M, Single B, Castoldi AF, Kühnle S, Nicotera P. Intracellular ATP concentration: a switch in the decision between apoptosis and necrosis. J Exp Med. 1997;185:1481–6.
93. Leist M, Auer-Barth S, Wendel A. Tumor necrosis factor production in the perfused mouse liver and its pharmacological modulation by methylxanthines. J Pharmacol Exp Ther. 1996;276:968–76.
94. Gantner F, Leist M, Küsters S, Vogt K, Volk D, Tiegs G. T cell stimulus-induced crosstalk between lymphocytes and liver macrophages results in augmented cytokine release. Exp Cell Res. 1996;229:137–46.
95. Wendel A. Biochemical pharmacology of inflammatory liver injury in mice. Meth Enzymol. 1990;186:675–80.

96. Jilg S, Barsig J, Leist M, Küsters S, Volk H-D, Wendel A. Enhanced release of interleukin-10 and soluble tumor necrosis factor receptors as novel principles of methylxanthine action in murine models of endotoxic shock. J Pharmacol Exp Ther. 1996;278:421–31.
97. Tiegs G, Niehörster M, Wendel A. Leukocyte alterations do not account for hepatitis induced by endotoxin or TNF-alpha in galactosamine-sensitized mice. Biochem Pharmacol. 1990;40: 1317–22.
98. Gantner F, Leist M, Jilg S, German PG, Freudenberg MA, Tiegs G. Tumor necrosis factor-induced hepatic DNA fragmentation as an early marker of T cell-dependent liver injury in mice. Gastroenterology. 1995;109:166–76.
99. Nagata S, Golstein P. The Fas death factor. Science. 1995;267:1449–55.
100. Stanger BZ. Looking beneath the surface: the cell death pathway of Fas/APO-1 (CD95). Mol Med. 1996;2:7–20.
101. Oehm A, Behrmann I, Kalk W et al. Purification and molecular cloning of the APO-1 cell surface antigen, a member of the tumour necrosis factor/nerve growth factor receptor family. J Biol Chem. 1992;267:10709–15.
102. Yonehara S, Ishii A, Yonehara M. A cell-killing monoclonal antibody (anti-Fas) to a cell surface antigen co-downregulated with the receptor of tumor necrosis factor. J Exp Med. 1989;169: 1747–56.
103. Boldin MP, Goncharov TM, Goltsev YV, Wallach D. Involvement of MACH, a novel MORT1/ FADD-interacting protease, in Fas/APO-1- and TNF receptor-induced cell death. Cell. 1996;85: 803–15.
104. Muzio M, Chinnaiyan AM, Kischkel FC et al. FLICE, a novel FADD-homologous ICE/CED-3-like protease, is recruited to the CD95 (Fas/APO-1) death-inducing signaling complex. Cell. 1996;85:817–27.
105. Ogasawara J, Watanabe-Fukunaga R, Adachi M et al. Lethal effect of the anti-fas antibody in mice. Nature. 1993;364:806–9.
106. Künstle G, Leist M, Uhlig S et al. ICE-protease inhibitors block murine liver injury and apoptosis caused by CD95 or TNF-alpha. Immunol Lett. 1997;55:5–10.
107. French LE, Hahne M, Viard I et al. Fas and Fas ligand in embryos and adult mice: ligand expression in several immune-privileged tissues and coexpression in adult tissues characterized by apoptotic cell turnover. J Cell Biol. 1996;133:335–43.
108. Strand S, Hofmann WJ, Hug H et al. Lymphocyte apoptosis induced by CD95 (APO-1/Fas) ligand expressing tumor cells – a mechanism of immune evasion? Nature Med. 1996;2:1361–6.
109. Benedetti A, Jezequel AM, Orlandi F. A quantitative evaluation of apoptotic bodies in rat liver. Liver. 1988;8:172–7.
110. Adachi M, Suematsu S, Kondo T et al. Targeted mutation in the Fas gene causes hyperplasia in peripheral lymphoid organs and liver. Nature Genet. 1995;11:294–300.
111. Rensing-Ehl A, Frei K, Flury R et al. Local Fas/APO-1 (CD95) ligand-mediated tumor cell killing in vivo. Eur J Immunol. 1995;25:2253–8.
112. Gantner F, Küsters S, Wendel A, Hatzelmann A, Schudt C, Tiegs G. Protection from T cell-mediated murine liver failure by phosphodiesterase inhibitors. J Pharmacol Exp Ther. 1997; 280:53–60.
113. Redondo C, Flores I, Gonzalez A et al. Linomide prevents the lethal effect of anti-Fas antibody and reduces Fas-mediated ceramide production in mouse hepatocytes. J Clin Invest. 1996;98: 1245–52.
114. Leist M, Wendel A. Tunicamycin potently inhibits tumor necrosis factor-induced hepatocyte apoptosis. Eur J Immunol. 1995;292:201–4.
115. Ni R, Tomita Y, Matsuda K et al. Fas-mediated apoptosis in primary cultured mouse hepatocytes. Exp Cell Res. 1994;215:332–7.
116. Los M, van de Craen M, Penning LC et al. Requirement of an ICE/CED-3 protease for Fas/ APO-1-mediated apoptosis. Nature. 1995;375:81–3.
117. Tewari M, Dixit VM. Fas- and tumor necrosis factor-induced apoptosis is inhibited by the poxvirus crmA gene product. J Biol Chem. 1995;270:3255–60.
118. Enari M, Hug H, Nagata S. Involvement of an ICE-like protease in fas-mediated apoptosis. Nature. 1995;375:78–81.
119. Kumar S, Lavin MF. The ICE family of cysteine proteases as effectors of cell death. Cell Death Differ. 1996;3:255–67.
120. Rouquet N, Pagès J-C, Molina T, Briand P, Joulin V. ICE inhibitor YVADcmk is a potent therapeutic agent against in vivo liver apoptosis. Curr Biol. 1996;6:1192–5.

121. Rodriguez I, Matsuura K, Ody C, Nagata S, Vassalli P. Systemic injection of a tripeptide inhibits the intracellular activation of CPP32-like proteases in vivo and fully protects mice against fas-mediated fulminant liver destruction and death. J Exp Med. 1996;184:2067–72.
122. Lacronique V, Mignin A, Fabre M et al. Bcl-2 protects from lethal hepatic apoptosis induced by an anti-Fas antibody in mice. Nature Med. 1996;2:80–5.
123. Rouquet N, Allemand I, Grimber G, Molina T, Briand P, Joulin V. Protection of hepatocytes from Fas-mediated apoptosis by a non-transforming SV40 T-antigen mutant. Cell Death Diff. 1996; 3:91–6.
124. Corcoran GB, Fix L, Jones DP. Contemporary issues in toxicology. Apoptosis: molecular control point in toxicity. Toxicol Appl Pharmacol. 1994;128:169–81.
125. Columbano A. Cell death: current difficulties in discriminating apoptosis from necrosis in the context of pathological processes in vivo. J Cell Biochem. 1995;58:181–90.
126. Sun DY, Jiang S, Zheng L, Ojcius DM, Young JD. Separate metabolic pathways leading to DNA fragmentation and apoptotic chromatin condensation. J Exp Med. 1994;179:559–68.
127. Tsukidate K, Yamamoto K, Snyder JW, Farber JL. Microtubule antagonists activate programmed cell death (apoptosis) in cultured rat hepatocytes. Am J Pathol. 1993;143:918–25.
128. Böe R, Gjertsen T, Vintermyr OK, Houge G, Lanotte M, Döskeland SO. The protein phosphatase inhibitor okadaic acid induces morphological changes typical of apoptosis in mammalian cells. Exp Cell Res. 1991;195:237–46.
129. Laskin DL, Pendino KJ. Macrophages and inflammatory mediators in tissue injury. Annu Rev Pharmacol Toxicol. 1995;35:655–77.
130. Cascales M, Alvarez A, Gasco P, Fernandez Simon L, Sanz N, Bosca L. Cocaine-induced liver injury in mice elicits specific changes in DNA ploidy and induces programmed death of hepatocytes. Hepatology. 1994;20:992–1001.
131. Pritchard DJ, Butler WH. Apoptosis – the mechanism of cell death in dimethyl-nitrosamine-induced hepatotoxicity. J Pathol. 1989;158:253–60.
132. Ray SD, Sorge CL, Kamendulis LM, Corcoran GB. Ca^{++}-activated DNA fragmentation and dimethylnitrosamine-induced hepatic necrosis: effects of Ca^{++}-endonuclease and poly(ADP-ribose) polymerase inhibitors in mice. J Pharmacol Exp Ther. 1992;263:387–94.
133. Goldin RD, Hunt NC, Clark J, Wickramasinghe SN. Apoptotic bodies in a murine model of alcoholic liver disease: reversibility of ethanol-induced changes. J Pathol. 1993;171:73–6.
134. Ledda-Columbano GM, Coni P, Curto M et al. Induction of two different modes of cell death, apoptosis and necrosis, in rat liver after a single dose of thioacetamide. Am J Pathol. 1991;139: 1099–109.
135. Nolan JP. Intestinal endotoxins as mediators of hepatic injury – an idea whose time has come again. Hepatology. 1989;10:887–91.
136. Kerr JFR. An electron-microscopic study of liver cell necrosis due to heliotrine. J Pathol. 1969; 97:557–62.
137. Czaja MJ, Xu J, Alt E. Prevention of carbon tetrachloride-induced rat liver injury by soluble tumor necrosis factor receptor. Gastroenterology. 1995;107:1849–54.
138. Leist M, Gantner F, Naumann H et al. Tumor necrosis factor-induced apoptosis during poisoning with hepatotoxins. Gastroenterology. 1997;112:923–34.

4
T cell-mediated experimental liver injury

G. TIEGS, S. KÜSTERS and G. KÜNSTLE

INTRODUCTION

T lymphocytes activated by either viral antigens or auto-antigens or by allogenic stimulation appear to be responsible for liver damage in all types of chronic active hepatitis or during liver graft rejection. Activated T cells exhibit direct cytotoxicity or release proinflammatory cytokines which mediate hepatocellular death. In viral hepatitis the cytotoxic $CD8^+$ T cell response seems to be restricted to lysis of virus-infected hepatocytes in acute self-limited disease[1,2], whereas disease activity in chronic active hepatitis is related to a T helper 1 (Th1)-like cytokine response of intrahepatic $CD4^+$ T cells[3–5]. Circumstantial evidence from experimental animal models argues for a pathogenic role of Th1 cells in organ-specific autoimmune diseases[6]. With respect to human autoimmune liver disease $CD4^+$ T cells are the predominant population of the liver-infiltrating T cells[7] and Th1-like cytokines correlating with transaminase levels have been detected in sections of pathological hepatic tissue[8]. Th1 cells release proinflammatory cytokines such as interferon-γ (IFNγ) or tumour necrosis factor-α (TNF).

Dysregulation and overexpression of TNF was shown to evoke hepatic failure in experimental shock models using lipopolysaccharides (LPS) from Gram-negative bacteria and liver sensitization by either killed bacteria or inhibition of hepatic transcription (reviewed in Reference 9). In these models, monocytes and macrophages are activated by LPS to release TNF[10]. Administration of soluble recombinant TNF itself was shown to cause hepatic failure in mice, but only following sensitization of the liver by transcriptional inhibition[11–14]. Transgenic mice expressing IFNγ in the liver develop liver injury resembling chronic active hepatitis. *In vitro*, IFNγ induces cell death of mouse hepatocytes which is accelerated by TNF[16]. From this observation, it was concluded that IFNγ as such is cytotoxic to hepatocytes.

We recently described three experimental mouse models of inflammatory liver injury. In all three models, the production of proinflammatory cytokines, such as TNF, depends on activated T cells. T cells were stimulated by either T cell receptor activating antibodies or by the bacterial superantigen staphylococcal enterotoxin

B (SEB). These T cell activators induce liver injury in immunocompetent mice sensitized by D-galactosamine (GalN)[17], i.e. an aminosugar known to selectively inhibit hepatic transcription as early as 0.5 h after injection[13]. In the third model, the T cell mitogenic plant lectin concanavalin A (Con A) induces liver injury in non-sensitized mice[18–20].

T CELL-DEPENDENT LIVER INJURY IN D-GALACTOSAMINE-SENSITIZED MICE

Experimental T cell shock in mice can be induced by administration of the 145 2C11 monoclonal antibody (mAb) directed against the murine CD3 molecule, i.e. the signal transducing moiety of the T cell receptor (TcR). Anti-CD3 mAbs have been shown to be immunosuppressive by inducing both T cell depletion and down-modulation of the CD3/TcR complex. These properties of the antibody led to the clinical use of human orthoclone T3 anti-CD3 mAb against allograft rejection in transplant recipients. The pathophysiological side-effects of orthoclone T3 are characterized by shock-like symptoms following the first injection of the antibody and represent a major limitation of orthoclone T3 treatment.

Intravenous administration of 10 μg of the 145 2C11 mAb to GalN-sensitized mice induced the release of cytokines, such as TNF, interleukin (IL)-2, IFNγ, and granulocyte macrophage colony-stimulating factor (GM-CSF) into the circulation of the animals. Severe liver injury was assessable within 8 h after intervention by determination of alanine aminotransferase (ALT), aspartate aminotransferase, and sorbitol dehydrogenase. Liver damage was prevented by polyclonal anti-mouse TNF antibodies. In order to verify the contribution of T cells to TNF production and liver injury, we administered anti-CD3 mAb to GalN-sensitized athymic nude mice. These mice, bearing only immature T lymphocytes, were completely resistant to GalN/anti-CD3 mAb, i.e. they failed to release TNF and to develop liver injury[17].

Morphological examination of livers from GalN/anti-CD3 mAb-treated mice showed pyknotic nuclear figures of swollen necrotic hepatocytes. Moreover, hyperchromatic nuclear membranes of parenchymal cells indicative of apoptotic cell death as well as shrunken apoptotic hepatocytes and numerous apoptotic bodies were seen. In contrast to necrotic alterations, morphological apoptotic features were already visible five hours after GalN/anti-CD3 challenge. Apoptotic or activation-induced cell death results from specific signalling in most cases including activation of an endonuclease that specifically cleaves double-stranded DNA internucleosomally[21]. This DNA fragmentation indeed occurred in murine livers following administration of GalN/anti-CD3 mAb and was identified as a 180 bp DNA ladder on an agarose gel. Cytosolic oligonucleosome-bound DNA fragments were quantified by an ELISA with a monoclonal anti-histone capture antibody and a monoclonal anti-DNA detection antibody. As in the case of the morphological alterations, DNA fragmentation preceded hepatocyte leakage (assessed by plasma ALT activities) by three hours. DNA fragmentation was completely abolished by pretreatment of mice with anti-TNF antibodies prior to GalN/anti-CD3 mAb challenge[17].

Bacterial superantigens such as staphylococcal enterotoxin B (SEB) activate T cells[22] by specific binding to both major histocompatibility complex Class II molecules of antigen-presenting cells and particular V_β segments of T cell receptors of a large subset of T cells. This massive T cell activation gives rise to the production of TNF and other cytokines sufficient to evoke lethal shock[23] and liver injury[17,24] in GalN-sensitized mice. We investigated whether hepatic apoptosis may also occur in this experimental model. Indeed, administration of SEB to GalN-sensitized mice induced the formation of hepatocyte hyperchromatic nuclear membranes and apoptotic bodies as well as DNA-fragmentation that preceded the release of ALT. Again, anti-TNF antibodies prevented DNA fragmentation and ALT release in GalN/SEB challenged mice[17].

CONCANAVALIN A-INDUCED T CELL-DEPENDENT LIVER INJURY IN MICE

Hallmarks of liver injury

The plant lectin Concanavalin A (Con A) mitogenically stimulates T lymphocytes *in vitro* by induction of cytokine synthesis. *In vivo*, intravenous injection of Con A at a dose ≥1.5 mg/kg resulted in a liver-specific injury in different mouse strains[18]. Liver specificity was explained by showing a selective binding of fluorescein isothiocyanate-labelled Con A to the endothelial surfaces of the liver sinusoids[19]. No specific staining was observed in pulmonary or renal tissue or any of the organs examined. Con A-induced hepatotoxicity was recognizable by morphological evaluation[19], oligonucleosomal DNA fragmentation (see Figures 1–3)[13,20] as well as by determination of highly elevated activities of plasma transaminases (see Figures 2 and 3) and sorbitol dehydrogenase[18]. A significant increase in DNA fragmentation was observed as early as 4 h following injection of 25 mg/kg Con A (Figure 2)[13]. Quantitative morphological examination showed a significantly enhanced number of apoptotic bodies 5 h after challenge[13]. Plasma transaminase activities were significantly increased after 8 h (Figures 2 and 3)[13] and showed maximum levels 16 h following Con A injection (Figures 2 and 3). Twenty-four hours after Con A challenge, liver injury parameters tended to decrease. This observation was most striking in the anti-TNF or anti-IFNγ antibody-protected groups (Figures 2 and 3, see below) and possibly indicates the beginning of liver regeneration. It is important to note that Con A induced this sequence of early apoptotic and late necrotic hepatocyte death in livers of non-sensitized mice. In contrast to the GalN models, neither hepatic transcription nor translation was inhibited by Con A until the onset of liver damage[13].

T cell dependence

The protective pharmacological intervention spectrum displayed a specificity for immunosuppressive drugs, such as cyclosporin A, FK 506 and dexamethasone, indicating a lymphocyte-mediated process[18]. Indeed, mouse strains lacking immunocompetent T lymphocytes, i.e. mice bearing the severe combined immunodeficiency syndrome (SCID mice) or athymic nude mice, were resistant towards Con A. Pretreatment of mice with Thy1.2 mAb which depleted 83% of all T cells of a BALB/c mouse conferred resistance towards Con A. Moreover, selective

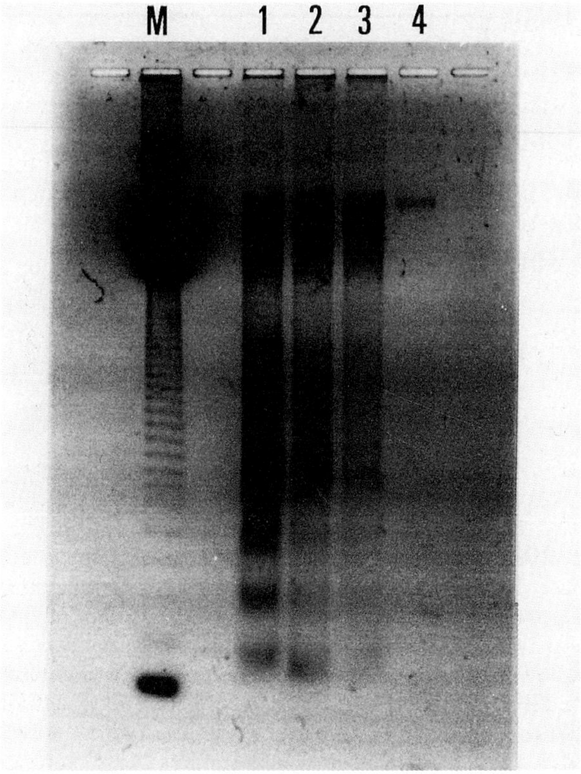

Figure 1. DNA fragmentation in livers of BALB/c mice 8 h after challenge with Con A. Sheep anti-muTNF polyclonal antiserum (50 μl/mouse), rabbit anti-muIFNγ polyclonal antiserum (200 μl/mouse), or control serum were injected iv 15 min prior to challenge. For semiquantitative determination of DNA fragmentation by analysing the pattern of low-molecular-weight DNA on an agarose gel, livers were perfused with cold buffer (50 mmol/L phosphate, 120 mmol/L NaCl, 10 mmol/L ethylenediaminetetra-acetic acid, pH 7.4) before excision. A 20% homogenate (in perfusion buffer) was prepared and centrifuged at 13 000*g* for 20 min. DNA was precipitated from the supernatant by addition of NaCl (5 mol/L)/ethanol, extracted by phenol/chloroform and again precipitation in ethanol. Subsequently, electrophoresis on a 1% agarose gel and ethidium bromide staining were performed. The $n \times 123$-bp molecular weight marker used for gel electrophoresis was from Gibco (Eggenstein, Germany). M, marker of 123-bp DNA ladder; 1, Con A only; 2, Con A pretreated with 200 μl anti-IFNγ antiserum per mouse; 3, Con A pretreated with 50 μl anti-TNF antiserum per mouse; 4; saline control

antibody-dependent depletion of T cell subpopulations indicated that $CD4^+$ T helper lymphocytes rather than $CD8^+$ cytotoxic T cells mediated Con A hepatotoxicity[18]. Immunohistochemical analyses of livers of Con A-treated mice showed that a large number of cells in the portal area were stained with an anti-mouse CD4 mAb whereas only a small number of cells exhibited the $CD8^+$ phenotype[25].

T helper cell activation depends on accessory cells, such as macrophages. In order to explore the nature of the accessory cells in the Con A hepatitis model, we performed *in-vitro* experiments with cocultures of murine adherent non-parenchymal liver cells containing 80–90% Kupffer cells (NPC) and primary murine lymph node cells (LNC). Each of the cell populations alone was scarcely

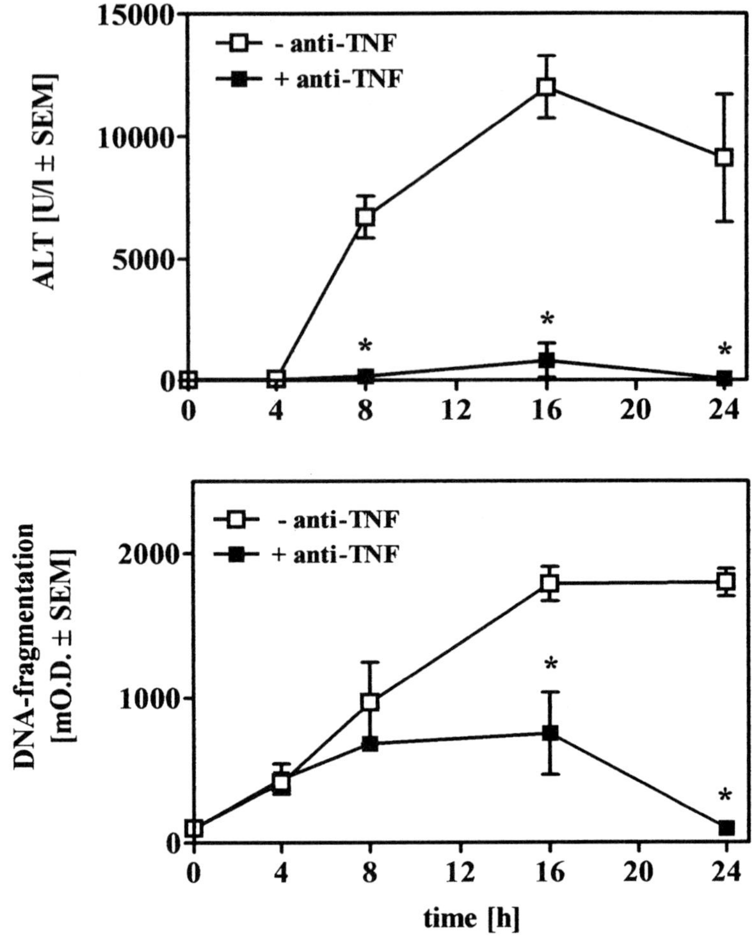

Figure 2. Time course of plasma ALT activity and hepatic DNA-fragmentation in mice after Con A challenge with and without pretreatment with anti-TNF antiserum. Plasma samples were taken at the times indicated for assessment of liver injury by measurement of plasma ALT activity. DNA fragmentation was measured by quantifying of cytosolic oligonucleosome-bound DNA using a cell death detection ELISA kit (Boehringer Mannheim, Mannheim, Germany). The 13000*g* supernatant from liver homogenates was used as antigen source in the sandwich ELISA with an anti-histone capture mAb and an anti-DNA detecting mAb coupled to peroxidase. The OD values of samples from Con A-challenged mice were compared with those samples from saline-treated control mice. Data are expressed as mean values ± SEM and were analysed by two-way analysis of variance (ANOVA) ($p < 0.05$) with the program INSTAT 2

activated by Con A as assessed by cytokine production. In contrast, cocultures of NPC and LNC produced substantial amounts of cytokines including the hepatotoxic mediators, TNF and IFNγ (see below)[19,26]. Concordantly, direct interactions between activated liver macrophages and lymphocytes were observed by electron microscopy 4[18] and 8 h (S. Angermüller and G. Tiegs, unpublished observation) after

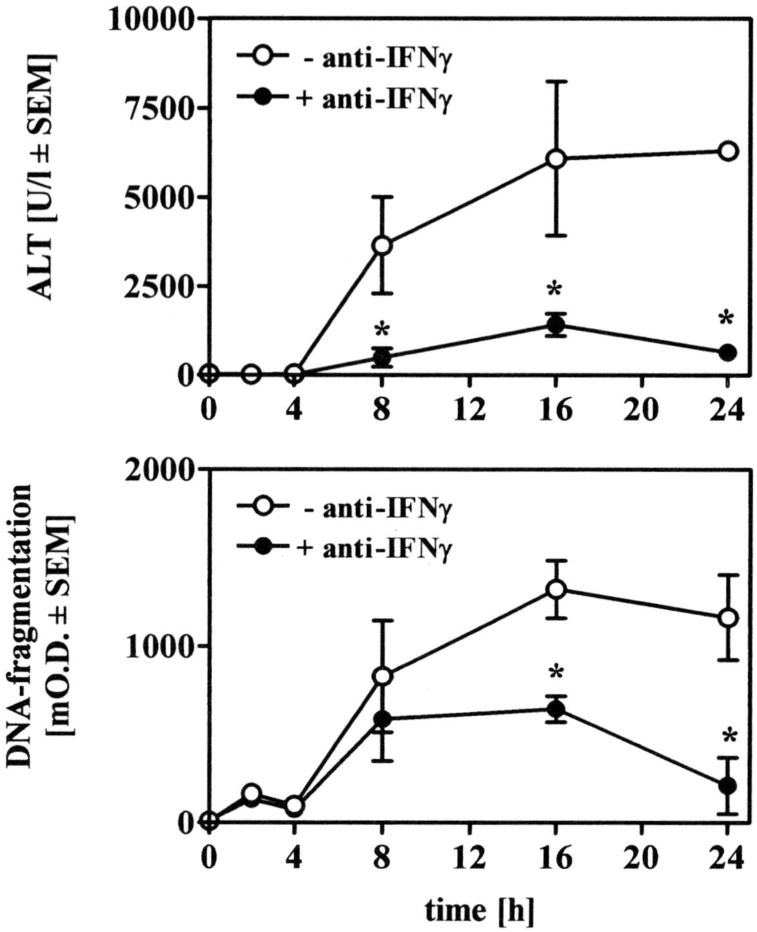

Figure 3. Time course of plasma ALT activity and hepatic DNA fragmentation in mice after Con A challenge with and without pretreatment with anti-IFNγ antiserum. For further details, see legend to Figure 2

Con A administration to mice, suggesting also that *in-vivo* macrophages provided accessory signals for Con A-induced T cell stimulation. However, at the onset of the pathogenic cascade, i.e. 15 min after intravenous injection, Con A preferentially bound to hepatic sinusoidal endothelial cells (SEC)[27]. *In vitro*, a Con A-specific $CD4^+$ T cell line displayed selective cytotoxicity towards syngenic primary murine SEC but not to Kupffer cells or fibroblasts in the presence of Con A. Although SEC functioned as accessory cells with respect to $CD4^+$ T cell-dependent TNF production in this *in-vitro* system, cytolysis of SEC was independent of TNF[27]. It was concluded from this study that SEC damage is likely to represent an early event in Con A-induced liver injury allowing the recruitment of T cells from the sinusoidal circulation and enabling the observed infiltration into hepatic

Table 1. Lack of induction of liver injury by simultaneous administration of TNF and IFNγ to mice

Treatment	ALT plasma activity (U/L)
GalN/TNF	9425±2450
TNF	43±2.0**
IFNγ	58±8.8**
TNF/IFNγ	44±1.9**

Plasma samples for determination of ALT activity were taken 8 h after iv injection of rmuTNF (10 μg/kg) or rmuIFNγ (50 μg/kg) in a total volume of 200 μl NaCl/0.1% HSA. GalN (700 mg/kg) was given ip in a total volume of 400 μl saline 15 min before TNF. Data are expressed as mean values±SEM; $n=3$; $**p<0.01$. Data were analysed by one-way analysis of variance (ANOVA) and subjected to Dunnett multiple comparisons test of the GalN/TNF-treated group against all other groups with the program INSTAT 2

tissue[25]. This conclusion was corroborated by the findings that inhibition of T cell recruitment to the extracellular matrix[28] as well as ICAM-1/LFA-1 blockade[29] prevented Con A-induced liver injury.

Role of TNF and IFNγ

Activation of T helper cells is usually associated with cytokine production. Indeed, the T-cell specific lymphokines, IL-2[18] and IL-4[30], as well as the cytokines, TNF, IFNγ, GM-CSF, IL-1, IL-6 and IL-10[19,20,25,30] were detectable in plasma of Con A-challenged mice. With the exception of IFNγ, the time courses of cytokine release showed a transient increase with maximal levels between 1 and 4h after Con A injection. IFNγ plasma levels steadily increased until 12h[20] and declined 24h[31] following Con A treatment. While IL-6 exhibited a protective effect towards Con A[25,31], TNF and IFNγ were identified as critical mediators of liver injury. Polyclonal anti-TNF as well as anti-IFNγ antibodies significantly protected mice from Con A-induced hepatic damage[19,20,25,31]. The time courses of liver injury with and without pretreatment with the respective antibodies are given in Figures 2 and 3. The results demonstrate that the antibodies prevented severe liver injury as detected by alanine aminotransferase, whereas a residual amount of DNA fragmentation, representing a very sensitive parameter of tissue damage, was still detectable after pretreatment with any of the antibodies (see also Figure 1) or with a combination of both[20]. Hence, it seems likely that additional signals beside TNF and IFNγ may contribute to Con A-induced hepatic apoptosis. Notably anti-IFNγ antibodies failed to prevent T cell infiltration into hepatic tissue[31], suggesting that the cytokines in fact exhibited direct hepatotoxic effects in the Con A model.

Further experiments showed that Con A-resistant nude mice failed to release TNF upon Con A administration. Concordantly, transfer of lymph node cells isolated from responder mice to nude resistant mice resulted in susceptibility of the nude mice towards Con A, i.e. to induction of TNF release and hepatotoxicity. These experiments demonstrated that the presence of immunocompetent T cells is necessary for Con A-stimulated TNF release *in vivo*[19].

Administration of soluble recombinant TNF to mice sensitized by transcriptional inhibitors such as GalN-induced liver injury (see Table 1) that was mediated by the TNFR60[14] but not by TNFR80 (data not shown). In the Con A model, TNF and IFNγ induced hepatic apoptosis and necrosis without the prerequisite of an overall transcriptional inhibition[13]. However, injection of soluble recombinant TNF alone or a combination of TNF and IFNγ into mice at doses even higher than those observed following Con A challenge, failed to induce liver injury (Table 1). Hence, a yet-unknown sensitization mechanism or additional cytotoxic factors are likely to be causally involved in Con A-induced liver injury.

Previous studies by Grell et al.[32] showed that cell lines fully resistant to the cytotoxic action of soluble TNF (sTNF) become highly susceptible upon activation by the transmembrane bioactive precursor of soluble TNF (mTNF). Moreover, mTNF cooperatively signals *via* both TNF receptors, i.e. TNFR60 and TNFR80, thereby leading to increased cellular responses compared with sTNF alone. We recently found in *in-vivo* experiments using transgenic mice deficient in sTNF but expressing a mutant non-cleavable form of mTNF[33] and by the use of TNFR60 and TNFR80 knockout mice, that mTNF (detectable in liver tissue by Western blot analysis following Con A challenge) was sufficient to mediate Con A-induced liver injury probably by activation of both TNF receptors (Küsters S, Tiegs G, Alexopoulou L et al., manuscript submitted for publication). These results corroborate the finding that metalloprotease inhibitors blocking the processing of mTNF and therefore the formation of sTNF aggravated hepatic injury induced by Con A[34]. These results provide an explanation for the ability of Con A to evoke TNF-dependent liver injury in the absence of transcriptional inhibition. Indirect support for a role of TNFR80 in human liver pathology was obtained in a recent study showing a strong up-regulation of hepatic TNFR80 expression in patients with chronic active hepatitis B virus infection[35].

Additional mediators

Perforin-deficient mice have been shown recently to be protected from liver injury induced by low doses of Con A[29]. At higher doses, these mice were sensitive towards Con A. These findings are consistent with results from our laboratory showing that perforin knockout mice[36] were as sensitive as the corresponding wild type towards liver injury induced by 25 mg/kg Con A (wildtype ALT: 546±398 U/L, perforin knockout ALT: 2090±974 U/L, $n=3$, not significant, tested by one-way analysis of variances). In contrast, mice which had received this latter dose of Con A were significantly protected from liver injury after pretreatment with anti-TNF or anti-IFNγ antibodies (see Figures 2 and 3). With respect to the residual hepatic DNA fragmentation observed following anti-TNF or anti-IFNγ antibody pretreatment of Con A-challenged mice, it seems worthwhile to further investigate the contribution of perforin and possibly other cytotoxic mediators of T cells[36] to hepatic apoptosis. However, our results and those from other laboratories suggest that TNF in its soluble and transmembrane form as well as IFNγ are the predominant mediators of Con A-induced liver injury.

PHARMACOLOGY OF T CELL-MEDIATED EXPERIMENTAL LIVER INJURY

Immunosuppressive drugs, such as cyclosporine A, FK 506, or dexamethasone, protected mice from T cell-mediated shock and liver injury inducible by either Con A[18], GalN/anti-CD3mAb[17], or GalN/SEB[23]. The non-steroidal anti-inflammatory drug indomethacin failed to prevent Con A hepatitis[18]. We recently found that the phosphodiesterase (PDE) inhibitors, motapizone (PDE3-selective) and rolipram (PDE4-selective), protected mice from Con A and GalN/SEB-induced liver injury at doses of 1–10 mg/kg. The protective effect correlated with an inhibition of TNF, IFNγ and IL-4 production, whereas circulating levels of the anti-inflammatory cytokine IL-10 were significantly increased[30]. These results correspond to earlier findings from LPS-models[37] and demonstrate that PDE inhibitors effectively attenuate an inflammatory T cell response *in vivo*, strongly suggesting a therapeutic potential for the treatment of T cell-related disease.

Acknowledgements

We thank Dr M. Schröter and Dr J. Tschopp, University of Lausanne, Institute of Biochemistry, Epalinges, Switzerland, for kindly providing the perforin knockout mice. We are indebted to Dr G. Adolf, Bender & Co., Vienna, Austria, for kindly providing TNF and IFNγ, and to Dr A. Wendel, University of Konstanz, Konstanz, Germany, for providing antisera that neutralize murine TNF or murine IFNγ, respectively. The work reviewed here was supported by the Deutsche Forschungsgemeinschaft, grants Ti 169/3-3 and Ti 169/4-1.

References

1. Ando K, Moriyama T, Guidotti LG et al. Mechanisms of class I restricted immunopathology. A transgenic mouse model of fulminant hepatitis. J Exp Med. 1993;178:1541–54.
2. Löhr HF, Gerken G, Schlicht HJ, Meyer zum Büschenfelde K-H, Fleischer B. Low frequency of cytotoxic liver-infiltrating T lymphocytes specific for endogenous processed surface and core proteins in chronic hepatitis B. J Infect Dis. 1993;168:1133–9.
3. Ferrari C, Mondelli MU, Penna A, Fiaccadori F, Chisari FV. Functional characterization of cloned intrahepatic, hepatitis B virus nucleoprotein-specific helper T cell lines. J Immunol. 1987;139: 539–44.
4. Löhr HF, Weber W, Schlaak J, Goergen B, Meyer zum Büschenfelde K-H, Gerken G. Proliferative response of CD4+ T cells and hepatitis B virus clearance in chronic hepatitis with or without hepatitis B e-minus hepatitis B virus mutants. Hepatology. 1995;22:61–8.
5. Napoli J, Bishop GA, McGuiness PH, Painter DM, McCaughan GW. Progressive liver injury in chronic hepatitis C infection correlates with increased intrahepatic expression of Th1-associated cytokines. Hepatology. 1996;24:759–65.
6. Liblau RS, Singer SM, McDevitt HO. Th1 and Th2 CD4+ T cells in the pathogenesis of organ-specific autoimmune diseases. Immunol Today. 1995;16:34–8.
7. Löhr HF, Schlaak JF, Gerken G, Fleischer B, Dienes H-P, Meyer zum Büschenfelde K-H. Phenotypical analysis and cytokine release of liver-infiltrating and peripheral blood T lymphocytes from patients with chronic hepatitis of different etiology. Liver. 1994;14:161–6.
8. Hussain JJ, Mustafa A, Gallati H, Mowat AP, Mieli-Vergani G, Vergani D. Cellular expression of tumor necrosis factor-α and interferon-γ in the liver biopsies of children with chronic liver disease. J Hepatol. 1994;21:816–21.

9. Tiegs G. Immunotoxicology of host response-mediated experimental liver injury. J Hepatol. 1994; 21:890–903.
10. Freudenberg MA, Keppler D, Galanos C. Requirement for lipopolysaccharide-responsive macrophages in galactosamine-induced sensitization to endotoxin. Infect Immunol. 1986;51: 891–5.
11. Tiegs G, Wolter M, Wendel A. Tumor necrosis factor is a terminal mediator in galactosamine/ endotoxin-induced hepatitis in mice. Biochem Pharmacol. 1989;38:627–31.
12. Leist M, Gantner F, Bohlinger I, Germann PG, Tiegs G, Wendel A. Murine hepatocyte apoptosis induced *in vitro* and *in vivo* by TNF-α requires transcriptional arrest. J Immunol. 1994;153: 1778–87.
13. Leist M, Gantner F, Bohlinger I, Tiegs G, Germann PG, Wendel A. Tumor necrosis factor-induced hepatocyte apoptosis precedes liver failure in experimental murine shock models. Am J Pathol. 1995;146:1220–34.
14. Leist M, Gantner F, Jilg S, Wendel A. Activation of the 55 kDa TNF receptor is necessary and sufficient for TNF-induced liver failure, hepatocyte apoptosis, and nitrite release. J Immunol. 1995; 154:1307–16.
15. Toyonaga T, Hino O, Sugai S et al. Chronic active hepatitis in transgenic mice expressing interferon-γ in the liver. Proc Natl Acad Sci USA. 1994;91:614–18.
16. Morita M, Watanabe Y, Akaike T. Protective effect of hepatocyte growth factor on interferon-gamma-induced cytotoxicity in mouse hepatocytes. Hepatology. 1995;21:1585–93.
17. Gantner F, Leist M, Jilg S, Germann PG, Freudenberg MA, Tiegs G. Tumor necrosis factor-induced hepatic DNA fragmentation as an early marker of T cell-dependent liver injury in mice. Gastroenterology. 1995;109:166–76.
18. Tiegs G, Hentschel J, Wendel A. A T-cell dependent experimental liver injury in mice inducible by concanavalin A. J Clin Invest. 1992;90:196–203.
19. Gantner F, Leist M, Lohse AW, Germann PG, Tiegs G. Concanavalin A-induced T cell-mediated hepatic injury in mice: the role of tumor necrosis factor. Hepatology. 1995;21:190–8.
20. Küsters S, Gantner F, Künstle G, Tiegs G. Interferon-γ plays a critical role in T cell-dependent liver injury in mice initiated by concanavalin A. Gastroenterology. 1996;111:462–71.
21. Wyllie AH. Glucocorticoid-induced thymocyte apoptosis is associated with endogenous endonuclease activation. Nature. 1980;284:555–6.
22. MacDonald HR, Baschieri S, Lees RK. Clonal expansion precedes anergy and death of $V_\beta 8^+$ peripheral T cells responding to staphylococcal enterotoxin B *in vivo*. Eur J Immunol. 1991;21: 1963–6.
23. Miethke T, Wahl C, Heeg K, Echtenacher B, Krammer PH, Wagner H. T cell-mediated lethal shock triggered in mice by the superantigen staphylococcal enterotoxin B: critical role of tumor necrosis factor. J Exp Med. 1992;175:91–8.
24. Nagaki M, Muto Y, Ohnishi H et al. Hepatic injury and lethal shock in galactosamine sensitized mice induced by the superantigen staphylococcal enterotoxin B. Gastroenterology. 1994;106: 450–8.
25. Mizuhara H, O'Neill E, Seki N et al. T cell activation-associated hepatic injury: mediation by tumor necrosis factor and protection by interleukin 6. J Exp Med. 1994;179:1529–37.
26. Gantner F, Leist M, Küsters S, Vogt K, Volk H-D, Tiegs G. T cell stimulus-induced crosstalk between lymphocytes and liver macrophages results in augmented cytokine release. Exp Cell Res. 1996;229:137–46.
27. Knolle PA, Gerken G, Löser E et al. Role of sinusoidal endothelial cells of the liver in concanavalin A-induced hepatic injury in mice. Hepatology. 1996;24: 824–9.
28. Hershkoviz R, Lider O, Bruck R, Aeed H, Greenspoon N, Halpern Z. Treatment of immune cell-mediated liver damage by nonpeptidic mimetics of the extracellular matrix-associated Arg-Gly-Asp epitope. J Hepatol. 1995;22:158–64.
29. Watanabe Y, Morita M, Akaike T. Concanavalin A induces perforin-mediated but not Fas-mediated hepatic injury. Hepatology. 1996;24:702–10.
30. Gantner F, Küsters S, Wendel A, Hatzelmann A, Schudt C, Tiegs G. Protection from T cell-mediated murine liver failure by phosphodiesterase inhibitors. J Pharmacol Exp Ther. 1997;280: 53–60.
31. Mizuhara H, Uno M, Seki N et al. Critical involvement of interferon gamma in the pathogenesis of T-cell activation-associated hepatitis and regulatory mechanisms of interleukin-6 for the manifestation of hepatitis. Hepatology. 1996;23:1608–15.

32. Grell M, Douni E, Wajant H et al. The transmembrane form of tumor necrosis factor is the prime activating ligand of the 80 kDa tumor necrosis factor receptor. Cell. 1995;83:793–802.
33. Douni E, Akassoglou K, Alexopoulou L et al. Transgenic and knockout analyses of the role of TNF in immune regulation and disease pathogenesis. J Inflamm. 1996;47:27–38.
34. Solorzano CC, Ksontini R, Pruitt JH et al. Involvement of 26-kDa cell-associated TNF-α in experimental hepatitis and exacerbation of liver injury with a matrix metalloproteinase inhibitor. J Immunol. 1997;158:414–19.
35. Marinos G, Naoumov NV, Rossol S et al. Tumor necrosis factor receptors in patients with chronic hepatitis B virus infection. Gastroenterology. 1995;108:1453–63.
36. Lowin B, Hahne M, Mattmann C, Tschopp J. Cytolytic T-cell cytotoxicity is mediated through perforin and Fas lytic pathway. Nature. 1994;370:650–2.
37. Jilg S, Barsig J, Leist M, Küsters S, Volk H-D, Wendel A. Enhanced induction of interleukin-10 and shedding of tumor necrosis factor receptors as possible protective principles of methylxanthines in murine models of endotoxic shock. J Pharmacol Exp Ther. 1996;278:421–31.

5
Lessons learned from animal models

A. W. LOHSE, S. KANZLER, P. KNOLLE and
K-H. MEYER ZUM BÜSCHENFELDE

INTRODUCTION: WHAT TO EXPECT FROM ANIMAL MODELS

In the study of experimental animals, questions as to the significance of animal models for human disease in general and for the particular disease of interest are paramount. Therefore, before embarking on animal studies, we have to ask what animal models can teach us, what are their opportunities and what are their limitations. None of the experimental animal diseases are ever an exact reflection of the human condition, be it in infectious processes, tumour development or autoimmune disease. However, this limitation is, in many respects, offset by the unique opportunity to study complex biological processes in the living organism that would never be attainable by *in-vitro* techniques. In a negative way, we are replacing *in-vitro* artefacts with 'animal artefacts'. With this in mind, however, we are then able to greatly enlarge our understanding of complex disease processes and test new therapeutic approaches by using animal models in a way that would never be possible by *in-vitro* studies on the one hand and clinical studies on the other.

What are the specific questions to be asked of animal models in the context of autoimmune hepatitis? They relate to principles of autoimmune disease in general, to liver-specific aspects of (auto-)immune reactions, and to cell-biological mechanisms of inflammation, cell death and fibrogenesis in the liver. Therefore, it is not only animal models of autoimmune hepatitis that require discussion in this context, but also other animal models of autoimmune disease as well as other models of inflammation, cell death and fibrogenesis.

ANIMAL MODELS OF AUTOIMMUNE DISEASE

Autoimmune disease processes can be induced in healthy animals by immunization in suitable adjuvants. Immunization in most models is performed using tissue-specific antigen extracts, such as myelin basic protein in the case of experimental autoimmune encephalomyelitis (EAE), collagen type II in the case of collagen arthritis (CA) or thyroglobulin in the case of experimental autoimmune thyroiditis

(EAT), but may also be induced with foreign antigens such as mycobacterium tuberculosis in the case of adjuvant arthritis (AA)[1]. All these models have in common the use of very strong adjuvant, which is best provided by complete Freund's adjuvant (CFA) as an emulsion of oils and mycobacteria with the respective antigen preparation. These models also have in common that, although they can be induced in various strains and species, there is a marked genetic component with some strains being completely resistant to disease induction and others being very susceptible[1,2]. Thus these models together demonstrate that an apparently healthy immune system can be induced by suitable (and strong) stimulation to mount a destructive immune response against self antigens leading to clinically overt disease, but genetic factors limit susceptibility to this phenomenon. This very much seems to reflect clinical observation in basically all autoimmune diseases: autoimmune diseases apparently arise in primarily healthy humans that are genetically susceptible. Patients, like these animal models, often carry MHC genes known to be associated with disease susceptibility, but MHC genes do not account for all the genetic risk profile. In the models of EAE and AA, for example, Fisher rats are resistant while Lewis rats are susceptible[2]. Both strains carry the same MHC. The difference in susceptibility in these strains is thought to be due to the different degree of genetically determined ability to secrete corticosteroids in response to stress.

Study of these animal models has further enlarged our understanding of the pathophysiology of autoimmune diseases and thus opened new therapeutic perspectives. In particular, the role of autoreactive CD4-positive antigen-specific T cells could be defined as the critical mediator of autoimmune disease in almost all disease models. Ben-Nun, Wekerle and Cohen in 1981 were the first to demonstrate that cloned activated myelin basic protein-specific T cells were able to induce EAE in naive animals[3]. Having identified the pathogenic agent, they were able to take their cue from microbiological principles of vaccination against disease by using attenuated agents of the disease as a vaccine protecting from the disease this agent normally causes: attenuating the disease-causing anti-MBP T cells by irradiation prevented disease induction but induced, in the vaccinated animals, a state of protection from subsequent attempts at disease induction, a principle therefore named T cell vaccination[4]. T cell vaccination has since been applied in a number of other animal models[5].

T cell vaccination has allowed us to study further principles of control mechanisms of autoreactive T cells operative both in the diseased and the healthy animal[6]. T cell vaccination induces two types of anti-T cell cellular immune responses, one specific for the vaccinating T cell clone, presumably anti-idiotypic, and one specific to the activation state of the vaccinating cell population, called anti-ergotypic[7–9]. The latter phenomenon was able to explain why only activated cells can vaccinate, which teleologically makes good sense since only activated cells are capable of inducing autoimmune disease and thus in need of a regulatory control. The major therapeutic potential probably lies in the anti-idiotypic response induced by T cell vaccination[9]. Further study of this phenomenon suggests that the variable region of the T cell receptor is the target of this response, making it possible to vaccinate with TCR-peptides or allowing DNA vaccination with TCR cDNA[10].

Transferring these therapeutic options to the clinic may still be a long way off, but initial studies have been very encouraging[11–13]. In particular, the studies by Zhang *et al.* in patients with multiple sclerosis have shown the feasibility of vaccination with specific anti-MBP T cell clones inducing specific deletion of the respective clonotypes from the peripheral immune system and apparent clinical benefit[13]. Exploring this approach further may in the future allow very specific and non-toxic intervention in autoimmune diseases.

EXPERIMENTAL AUTOIMMUNE HEPATITIS

Various animal models of autoimmune hepatitis have been described in the past and no standard model has really been established throughout the world[14]. Nonetheless, these models have very much in common and experimental differences appear to be minor.

Experimental hepatitis in rabbits was described by Meyer zum Büschenfelde and Kössling using immunization with heterologous (human) liver antigen preparation in CFA[15]. By using repeated immunizations, the histological picture of chronic active hepatitis could be induced[16]. These studies helped to identify the so-called liver-specific protein (LSP) as putative autoantigen in autoimmune liver diseases and characterize anti-LSP antibodies as markers of autoimmune hepatitis both in animals and in patients[17,18]. Although LSP was later identified as a relatively crude antigen mixture and anti-LSP antibodies are no longer in use, these studies have laid the basis for the identification of further and more specific autoantibody – antigen systems, in particular antibodies to the asialoglycoprotein receptor[19,20] and antibodies to a soluble liver antigen[21] whose molecular antigen has not yet been identified. Both these antibody systems have reached significant clinical relevance in the diagnosis of autoimmune hepatitis.

Cellular immune response can only be reliably studied in inbred animals necessitating the establishment of murine animal models of autoimmune hepatitis. This has been accomplished by a number of groups using similar preparations of crude liver antigens in CFA. The animal strain most susceptible to the models of experimental autoimmune hepatitis (EAH) is C57BL/6 mice[22]. Repeated intramuscular immunizations have been described by several groups to induce a picture of chronic hepatitis in these animals[22,23]. We have been able to facilitate induction of EAH by introducing intraperitoneal immunization[24]. A single immunization is sufficient to induce a prolonged hepatic inflammatory disease process, presumably by increasing the local immune response to the disease-relevant autoantigen(s) and thus circumventing peripheral immunoregulatory mechanisms[24,25]. This is illustrated by Figures 1 and 2. Figure 1 shows the difference in disease severity depending on the mode of disease induction, where it is clearly demonstrated that intraperitoneal immunization is much more potent than other modes of immunization. Figure 2 depicts the proliferative T cell response of lymphocytes isolated from the liver, the spleen and the cervical lymph node after ip immunization. It can be seen that the local immune response as found in liver and spleen (which should both be viewed as draining lymphoid compartments) is much more pronounced than the response in the cervical lymph node.

Several groups have shown EAH to be a T cell-mediated disease. This is demonstrated most clearly by passive transfer experiments[22,24]. It is the CD4 population

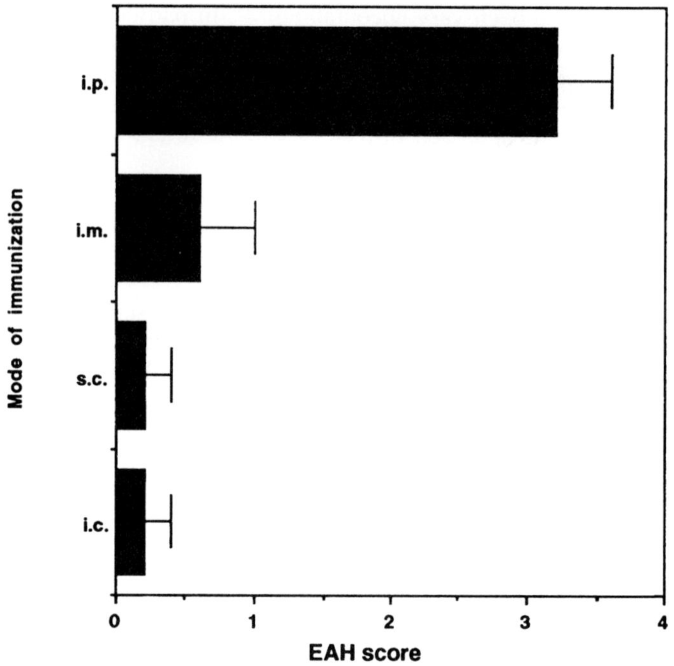

Figure 1. Hepatitis scores after a single immunization with S-100 antigen in CFA. EAH was induced by immunization with freshly prepared syngeneic S-100 (2.5 mg/animal) in CFA and animals sacrificed 21 days later to assess histological disease severity

that appears to mediate the disease. Furthermore, autoantibodies arise very late in the course of the disease and tend to increase in titre well beyond histological improvement of the disease process[26].

As in all the other models of induced autoimmune disease, EAH is a transient disease process with spontaneous recovery about three to four weeks after the last immunization[24]. This has led us to study immunoregulatory phenomena in the model of EAH. We could observe that while disease induction was associated with a marked T cell response to liver antigens and both an antigen-specific and an antigen-non-specific helper response, at the peak of disease activity (which at the same time is of course the beginning of recovery), there was a marked suppressive activity, again both antigen-specific and antigen-non-specific[27]. This was associated with marked non-responsiveness to *in-vivo* administration of another strong immunogen, tetanus toxoid[27].

Very similar observations could be made in patients with autoimmune hepatitis, although here the spontaneous course of the disease cannot be followed as withholding therapy would be unethical. Nonetheless, we could clearly demonstrate both antigen-specific and antigen-non-specific suppression in patients with AIH in remission. Even more impressively, there was almost complete non-

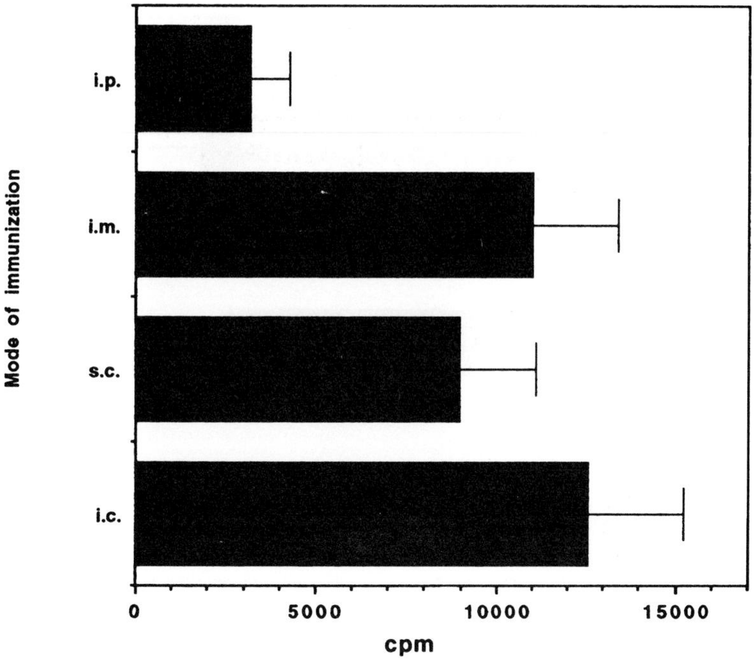

Figure 2. Systemic (cervical lymph node) T-cell response to liver autoantigens after different modes of immunization

responsiveness to a tetanus toxoid booster immunization in patients with active untreated autoimmune hepatitis, suggesting generalized immunosuppression, presumably as an attempt by the immune system to correct its own aberrant autoimmune response[28]. This ability of the immune system to at least partly correct harmful autoimmune reactions may account for the often spontaneously fluctuating course of autoimmune hepatitis that can be observed in many patients, as well as long-lasting complete remissions even after cessation of all immunosuppressive drugs[29]. The presence of such regulatory control mechanisms is furthermore encouraging when planning to establish specific immunotherapy that aims at augmenting these regulatory responses in order to regain homeostasis.

T cell vaccination was mentioned above as a new prospect of specific immunotherapy. We have recently extended the study of T cell vaccination to the model of EAH and found it to be effective in suppressing the disease[30]. This underlines the regulatory cycles available to the immune system in autoimmune hepatitis, which could, when suitably stimulated, correct the aberrant autoimmune response in order to regain physiological self-tolerance, and it opens the prospect of specific immunotherapy in clinical autoimmune hepatitis.

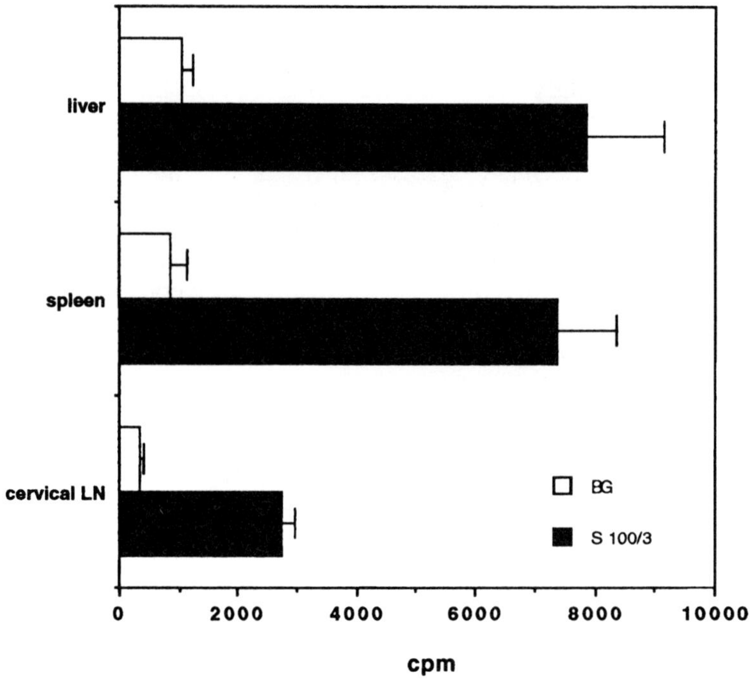

Figure 3. T-cell response in the liver, spleen and cervical lymph node after intraperitoneal immunization. EAH was induced by immunization with syngeneic S-100 proteins i.p. and animals sacrificed on day 10 to remove liver, spleen and cervical lymph nodes. Lymphocytes were isolated by density centrifugation in the case of the liver and by simple cell meshes for spleen and lymph nodes, and tested in a standard T cell proliferation assay against the small molecular weight fraction of the S-100 antigen preparation

ANIMAL MODELS OF HEPATIC INJURY, CELL DEATH AND FIBROGENESIS

Animal models of liver damage other than autoimmune-mediated liver damage can teach us various aspects of hepatocyte damage, repair mechanisms and the most detrimental hepatic repair mechanism, fibrogenesis. Two types of model appear of particular interest in this context: firstly, the model of Concanavalin A-induced T cell-dependent hepatic injury (Con A hepatitis)[31], which is discussed in detail in earlier chapters, and secondly the model of carbon tetrachloride-induced fibrogenesis.

Con A hepatitis is induced in susceptible strains of mice by intravenous injection of very large amounts of Con A[31]. Like autoimmune disease models, susceptibility between strains varies, thus demonstrating a genetic component in a non-autoimmune liver disease model. The liver injury is primarily mediated by CD4+ T lymphocytes with cytotoxic activity, similar to other autoimmune disease models[31].

Cytokines appear to play an essential role in mediation of the liver injury as blockade of TNFα and IFNγ can prevent disease or ameliorate the course[32]. Interleukin 10 appears to be protective while interleukin 12 is detrimental in this model. An intriguing aspect is why the liver is injured in this model while other organs primarily in contact with the intravenously injected Con A, such as the lungs or the gut, appear to remain healthy. Preferential binding of Con A to the hepatic sinusoidal endothelial cells[32] and rapid killing of the endothelial cells appears to be the first step in this model, underlining the unique role of hepatic sinusoidal endothelial cells (SEC) in immune mechanisms in the liver[33].

This model has also focused attention on the role of hepatic SEC in antigen presentation. Hepatic SEC were recently shown by us to be very effective antigen-presenting cells[34]. This raises very important questions as SEC together with Kupffer cells, which are also capable of effective antigen presentation, are the cells primarily in contact with circulating lymphocytes. These cells may be of primary importance in inducing an autoimmune reaction in the liver. However, antigen presentation in the liver appears to normally favour a state of immunological tolerance as demonstrated by experiments comparing intraportal with intravenous antigen challenge. We thus need to explain the factors that normally favour tolerance induction in the hepatic microenvironment, but that may be disturbed in autoimmune liver diseases. Interleukin 10, which is produced locally by Kupffer cells[35], may be an important downregulator of antigen presentation in the liver, and it appears that absence of interleukin 12 might be critical. These studies have focused on *in-vitro* isolated cell populations taking their cues from animal models, and it is probably necessary to go back to the animal to study the *in-vivo* significance before drawing conclusions about human disease.

The model of CCl_4 deserves mention in this context as it has, more than any other approach, helped to elucidate the mediators of fibrogenesis, and has in particular defined transforming growth factor β (TGFβ) as the most important fibrogenetic factor in the liver[36,37]. Fibrogenesis is an important feature of autoimmune hepatitis, a condition in which subclinical development of cirrhosis is often observed. We have recently looked for TGFβ in autoimmune hepatitis and found very high serum levels in active disease that normalized in remission. Furthermore, production of TGFβ in the peripheral blood was normal but expression in the liver was very high as measured by immunohistology and *in-situ* hybridization. It is particularly intriguing that TGFβ is at the same time a potent immunoinhibitory cytokine. TGFβ may thus account partly for the spontaneous immunosuppression observed in AIH, as described above, as well as the rapid fibrogenesis seen. As fibrosis is the ultimate limitation of liver regeneration in autoimmune hepatitis, study of this final pathway of inflammatory liver disease and therapeutic intervention at this point will remain of interest also in AIH, and we will continue to observe models of fibrogenesis, such as CCl_4, as well as, for example, bile duct ligation or schistosomiasis.

TRANSGENIC MOUSE MODELS

The past few years have seen rapid progress in the study of human disease in animals by use of transgenic and knock-out models. At present, there is no model of autoimmune hepatitis in transgenic animals but there are a number of models with major relevance to the study of autoimmune hepatitis and others are currently being developed.

For a number of years, Chisari and co-workers have been studying transgenic animal models of hepatitis B[38]. In a way, these are autoimmune liver disease models as the hepatitis B antigens expressed in hepatocytes of transgenic mice can be considered to be liver specific neoantigen. Under normal conditions, these mice are tolerant to their new liver autoantigen, as would be expected for an antigen present in fetal life. However, passive transfer of hepatitis B-specific T cell lines can induce hepatitis in these animals. These studies have helped to study the *in-vivo* conditions of hepatocyte damage in an antigen-specific T cell-mediated hepatitis model. Both perforin-mediated cytotoxicity and apoptosis were shown to play a role in this model, while antiviral activity was linked to interferon γ production[38].

As explained elsewhere in this book, Arnold *et al.* have described very revealing transgenic mouse experiments that give us major insight into the mechanisms of tolerance induction in the peripheral immune system[39]. They produced transgenics overexpressing an allo MHC molecule under various promoters and crossed these animals with mice transgenic for the T cell receptor specifically reactive with this allo MHC. When using liver-specific promoters (albumin and CRP), alloreactive T cells could be detected but the CD8 molecule as well as the TCR were down-regulated. When using the inducible CRP promoter with only minimal basal expression of the transgene, down-regulation was not observed, but, upon up-regulation of transgene expression by induction of the CRP promoter, TCR and CD8 down-regulation were again observed, demonstrating mechanisms of extra-thymic tolerance induction in otherwise healthy mice[40]. Extending these studies to other transgene-expressing sites (skin, central nervous system), this group beautifully demonstrated the presence of multiple levels of tolerance induction present beyond the thymus[39]. The mechanisms of this tolerance induction remain open to future study. Impressively though, the system appears to be very strongly biased towards tolerance, as all these models induced tolerance at various levels. It thus remains intriguing to speculate how tolerance can be broken as it is broken in patients with autoimmune diseases.

Future studies of autoimmune hepatitis in animal models will have to go further along these roads. We are thus currently developing various models of immune mechanisms in the liver using transgene technology. We are constructing transgenics overexpressing the 60-kDa heat-shock protein, which is much more immunogenic than the MHC molecule studied by Arnold *et al.* Furthermore, we have murine as well as bacterial HSP60, thus allowing comparison of the effects of over-expression of the self-homologue with the foreign antigen, and also allowing study of the effect of autoimmunization using CFA, which includes mycobacterial HSP60. On the other hand, we are trying to characterize the role of cytokines, in particular fibrogenetic factors, in autoimmune hepatitis by constructing mice with selective and inducible overexpression of TGFβ and platelet-derived growth factor (PDGF) in the liver. Induction of disease models, such as EAH or CCl_4, in these transgenics will be helpful in further disecting the mechanisms of autoimmune liver disease.

CONCLUSIONS

Each animal model can only help us to understand certain aspects of the complexity of human disease, and autoimmune hepatitis is no exception to this rule. The multitude of models available and the new technological advances have, however, already provided major advances in the analysis of the mechanisms of autoimmune hepatitis and, most importantly, have opened the perspective of specific immunotherapy. Transgenic technology is expected to highlight the importance of *in-vivo* animal studies and will rapidly advance our knowledge of disease mechanisms, including autoimmune hepatitis. While some observations have already been transferred to clinical studies, transferring new therapeutic approaches from the animal house to the bedside is still a long way off, but it will most certainly happen.

References

1. Cohen I, Miller A. Guidebook to Animal Models for Autoimmune Diseases. Orlando: Academic Press; 1994.
2. Arnon R. Experimental allergic encephalomyelitis – susceptibility and suppression. Immunol Rev. 1981;55:5.
3. Ben-Nun A, Wekerle H, Cohen IR. The rapid isolation of clonable antigen-specific T lymphocyte lines capable of mediating autoimmune encephalomyelitis. Eur J Immunol. 1981;11:195–9.
4. Ben-Nun A, Wekerle H, Cohen IR. Vaccination against autoimmune encephalomyelitis with T lymphocyte lines reactive against myelin basic protein. Nature. 1981;292:60–1.
5. Cohen IR, Ben-Nun A, Holoshitz J, Maron R, Zerubavel R. Vaccination against experimental diseases with lines of autoimmune T lymphocytes. Immunol Today. 1983;4:227–30.
6. Lohse AW, Cohen IR. Immunoregulation: studies of physiological and therapeutic autoreactivity by T cell vaccination. Springer Semin Immunopathol. 1992;14:179–86.
7. Lider O, Reshef T, Beraud E, Ben-Nun A, Cohen IR. Anti-idiotypic network induced by T cell vaccination against experimental autoimmune encephalomyelitis. Science. 1988;239:181–3.
8. Lohse AW, Mor F, Karin N, Cohen IR. Control of experimental autoimmune encephalomyelitis by T cells responding to activated T cells. Science. 1989;244:820–2.
9. Lohse AW, Cohen IR. Mechanisms of resistance to autoimmune disease induced by T cell vaccination. Autoimmunity. 1991;9:119–21.
10. Vandenbark AA, Hashim G, Offner H. Immunization with a synthetic T-cell receptor V-region peptide protects against experimental autoimmune encephalomyelitis. Nature. 1989;341:541–4.
11. Hafler D, Cohen IR, Benjamin DS, Weiner HL. T cell vaccination in multiple sclerosis: a preliminary report. Clin Immunol Immunopathol. 1992;62:307–13.
12. Lohse AW, Bakker N, Hermann E, Poralla T, Jonker M, Meyer zum Büschenfelde K-H. Induction of an anti-vaccine response by T cell vaccination in patients and non-human primates. J Autoimmun. 1993;1:121–8.
13. Zhang J, Medaer R, Stinissen P, Hafler D, Raus J. MHC-restricted depletion of human myelin basic protein-reactive T cells by T cell vaccination. Science. 1993;261:1451–4.
14. Lohse AW, Meyer zum Büschenfelde KH. Experimental hepatitis. In: Cohen IR, Miller A, eds. Autoimmune Disease Models: A Guidebook. San Diego: Academic Press; 1994:191–9.
15. Kössling FK, Meyer zum Büschenfelde KH. Zur Indukton einer aktiven chronischen Hepatitis durch heterologe Leberproteine. Virchows Arch Path Anat. 1968;345:365–76.
16. Meyer zum Büschenfelde KH, Miescher PA. Liver-specific antigens, purification and characterization. Clin Exp Immunol. 1972;10:89–102.
17. Meyer zum Büschenfelde KH, Knolle J, Berger J. Celluläre Immunreaktionen gegenüber homologen leberspezifischen Antigenen (HLP) bei chronischen Leberentzündungen. Klin Wochenschr. 1974;52:246–8.
18. Jensen DM, McFarlane IG, Portmann B et al. Detection of antibodies directed against a liver-specific membrane lipoprotein in patients with acute and chronic active hepatitis. N Engl J Med. 1978;299:1–7.

19. McFarlane IG, McFarlane BM, Major GN et al. Identification of the hepatic asialoglycoprotein receptor (hepatic lectin) as a component of liver specific membrane lipoprotein (LSP). Clin Exp Immunol. 1984;55:347–54.
20. Treichel U, Poralla T, Hess G, Manns M, Meyer zum Büschenfelde KH. Autoantibodies to human asialoglycoprotein receptor in autoimmune-type chronic active hepatitis. Hepatology. 1990;11: 606–12.
21. Manns M, Gerken G, Kyriatsoulis A, Staritz M, Meyer zum Büschenfelde K-H. Characterization of a new subgroup of autoimmune chronic active hepatitis by autoantibodies against a soluble liver antigen. Lancet. 1987;i:292–4.
22. Mori Y, Mori T, Yoshida H et al. Study of cellular immunity in experimental autoimmune hepatitis in mice. Clin Exp Immunol. 1984;57:85–92.
23. Kuriki J, Murakami H, Kakumu S et al. Experimental autoimmune hepatitis in mice after immunization with syngeneic liver proteins together with the polysaccharide of Klebsiella pneumoniae. Gastroenterology. 1983;84:596–603.
24. Lohse AW, Manns M, Dienes HP, Meyer zum Büschenfelde K-H, Cohen IR. Experimental autoimmune hepatitis: disease induction, time course and T-cell reactivity. Hepatology. 1990;11:24–30.
25. Lohse AW, Knolle P, Meyer zum Büschenfelde KH. Mode of immunization and T-cell reactivity to liver autoantigens in the induction of experimental autoimmune hepatitis. J Hepatol. 1995; 23(Suppl. 1):130.
26. Lohse AW, Brunner S, Kyriatsoulis A, Manns M, Meyer zum Büschenfelde K-H. Autoantibodies in experimental autoimmune hepatitis. J Hepatol. 1992;14:48–53.
27. Lohse AW, Meyer zum Büschenfelde KH. Remission of experimental autoimmune hepatitis is associated with increased antigen-specific and non-specific immunosuppression. Clin Exp Immunol. 1993;94:163–73.
28. Lohse AW, Kögel M, Meyer zum Büschenfelde KH. Evidence for spontaneous immunosuppression in autoimmune hepatitis. Hepatology. 1995 [In press].
29. Johnson PJ, McFarlane IG, Eddleston ALWF. The natural course and heterogeneity of autoimmune-type chronic active hepatitis. Semin Liver Dis. 1991;11(3):187–96.
30. Lohse AW, Waldmann C, Meyer zum Büschenfelde KH. Suppression of experimental autoimmune hepatitis by T cell vaccination. Hepatology. 1994;20:144A.
31. Tiegs G, Hentschel J, Wendel A. A T cell-dependent experimental liver injury in mice inducible by concanavalin A. J Clin Invest. 1992;90:196–203.
32. Gantner F, Leist M, Lohse AW, Germann PG, Tiegs G. Concanavalin A-induced T cell-mediated hepatic injury: the role of tumor necrosis factor. Hepatology. 1995;21:190–8.
33. Knolle P, Löser E, Gerken G, Meyer zum Büschenfelde K-H, Lohse A. Role of sinusoidal endothelial cells of the liver in Concanavalin A induced hepatic injury in mice. Hepatology. 1996; 24:824–30.
34. Lohse A, Knolle P, Bilo K et al. Antigen presenting function and B7 expression of murine sinusoidal endothelial cells and Kupffer cells. Gastroenterology. 1996;110:1175–81.
35. Knolle P, Schlaak J, Uhrig A, Kempf P, Meyer zum Büschenfelde K-H, Gerken G. Human Kupffer cells secrete IL-10 in response to lipopolysaccharide (LPS) challenge. J Hepatol. 1995;22:226–9.
36. Czaja MJ, Weiner FR, Flanders KC et al. In vitro and in vivo association of transforming growth factor-β1 with hepatic fibrosis. J Cell Biol. 1989;108:2477–84.
37. Nakatsukasa H, Nagy P, Evarts RP, Hsia C-C, Marsden E, Thorgeirsson SS. Cellular distribution of transforming growth factor-β1 and procollagen types I, III, and IV transcripts in carbon tetrachloride-induced rat liver fibrosis. J Clin Invest. 1990;85:1833–43.
38. Chisari FV. Hepatitis B virus transgenic mice: models of viral immunobiology and pathogenesis. Curr Top Microbiol Immunol. 1996;206:149–73.
39. Arnold B, Schönrich G, Hämmerling GJ. Multiple levels of peripheral tolerance. Immunol Today. 1993;14:12–14.
40. Ferber I, Schönrich G, Schenkel J, Mellor AL, Hämmerling G, Arnold B. Levels of peripheral T cell tolerance induced by different doses of tolerogen. Science. 1994;263:674–6.

Section II
Clinical aspects

6
Genetic aspects of autoimmune liver diseases

E. L. KRAWITT, R. J. ALBERTINI and P. DONALDSON

INTRODUCTION

To better understand the aetiology and pathogenesis of autoimmune liver diseases from a genetic point of view as related to extrahepatic manifestations, a number of factors must be considered. These include, but are not limited to, the following:

(1) Familial autoimmune liver disease is not common.

(2) Autoimmune liver disease does occur in families marked by a variety of autoimmune diseases.

(3) Extrahepatic disorders occur frequently in patients with autoimmune liver diseases, but vary depending on the type of autoimmune liver disease.

(4) Autoantibodies occur in patients and in first-degree relatives of patients with autoimmune liver diseases, although the pattern of autoantibodies varies depending on the type of autoimmune liver disease.

(5) The same autoantibodies may occur in patients with other autoimmune disorders and their first-degree relatives.

(6) Autoimmune liver diseases are associated with specific HLA phenotypes and genotypes; the HLA associations vary depending on the type of autoimmune liver disease.

(7) The HLA associations of extrahepatic manifestations may not correspond to those found in specific autoimmune liver diseases.

When considering these extrahepatic manifestations, perhaps the most striking association is that of primary sclerosing cholangitis (PSC) and non-specific ulcerative colitis. It is estimated that 60–70% of cases of PSC occur in association with non-specific ulcerative colitis. Ulcerative colitis is seen less frequently with autoimmune hepatitis (AIH). The occurrence of ulcerative colitis in primary biliary cirrhosis (PBC) is rare. PSC and ulcerative colitis both have a high prevalence of the relatively specific perinuclear antineutrophil cytoplasmic antibodies (pANCA). The HLA associations, however, differ considerably between these two diseases.

EXTRAHEPATIC MANIFESTATIONS OF AUTOIMMUNE LIVER DISEASES

Associated diseases

If we consider human autoimmune diseases to fall within a spectrum ranging from non-organ specific at one end to organ-specific at the other, autoimmune liver diseases lie somewhere in the middle, as they are confined for the most part to the liver, but the autoantibodies are generally non-specific. Nevertheless, AIH, PBC and PSC can be associated with a number of extrahepatic manifestations and diseases. Some of these manifestations and diseases are characterized by sex imbalances, as are the autoimmune liver diseases wherein PBC and AIH have a female preponderance, which is rather marked in PBC, while PSC has a less marked male preponderance.

Diseases commonly seen with AIH include haemolytic anemia, idiopathic thrombocytopenic purpura, diabetes mellitus, thyroiditis and non-specific ulcerative colitis; other disorders are seen less frequently. PBC is often accompanied by Raynaud's syndrome, Sicca syndrome, scleroderma and its variant the CREST syndrome, rheumatoid arthritis, systemic lupus erythematosus and/or thyroiditis. The major extrahepatic associations of PSC in addition to ulcerative colitis are pancreatitis and diabetes mellitus.

Autoantibodies

Type 1 or classical AIH is marked by circulating antibodies to nuclei and smooth muscle, the latter thought to be reflective of the more specific antiactin antibodies. Other antibodies described include those directed against a soluble liver antigen, a liver–pancreas protein, a plasma membrane sulphatide and the nuclear envelope proteins lamins A and C. On occasion, antimitochondrial antibodies occur concomitantly with these autoantibodies but the isolated presence of antimitochondrial antibodies signifies PBC except in the rare instances in which an overlap syndrome occurs.

The antimitochondrial antibody–primary biliary cirrhosis association probably reflects the most specific and most sensitive autoantibody association with autoimmune liver disease. Because of an almost explosive increase in our knowledge of the biochemistry of the mitochondrial 2-oxo acid dehydrogenase complexes (dominant antigen, dihydrolipoamide acetyltransferase component E2 of the pyruvate dehydrogenase complex), anti-M2 has become an important marker of PBC. Other autoantibodies found in PBC include those directed against nuclear membrane proteins including the nuclear pore complex, the lamin B receptor, gp210 and nucleoporin 62 which, although infrequently seen, does have a high specificity. Anti-gp210 may appear in antimitochondrial antibody-negative PBC and also appears to be higher in patients with associated arthritis.

Although it has been recognized for quite a while that antinuclear antibodies may appear in PSC, the discovery of a strong association of perinuclear anticytoplasmic antibodies (pANCA) with PSC has served to facilitate the diagnosis of and the tracking of the genetics of this disorder. Although characteristic of PSC, these autoantibodies have also been described in AIH. In some cases, they may merely reflect positive antinuclear antibodies measured in a neutrophil system but in others they represent true pANCA. Thus their prevalence is high not only in PSC but also in AIH. Ulcerative colitis, even in the absence of AIH or PSC, is the only other disease in which the prevalence of pANCA approaches that seen in PSC and AIH.

HLA ASSOCIATIONS OF AUTOIMMUNE LIVER DISEASES

Immunogenetic investigations of autoimmune liver diseases to date have included studies of the genes which encode the major histocompatibility (HLA), immunoglobulin (Ig) and T cell receptor (TCR) molecules. For the most part, however, these studies have been directed at the extremely polymorphic HLA loci on the short arm of chromosome 6. Only a limited number of studies have been performed examining immunoglobulin allotypes and TCR gene polymorphisms or variable region usage.

Classical (type 1) AIH is associated with the HLA DR3 serotype (which is found in linkage disequilibrium with HLA B8 and HLA A1) and with HLA DR4. HLA DR3-associated disease is more commonly found in the early onset, severe form of disease (often young girls and young women). HLA DR4 is more common in patients with the late-onset form of the disease and appears to be associated with a higher incidence of extrahepatic manifestations in Caucasian patients. In Japan, where HLA DR3 is extremely rare, the primary association is with HLA DR4.

Recent studies using PCR genotyping for HLA DRB, DQA and DQB have confirmed the serological studies and revealed a high frequency of the HLA DRB1*0301-DRB3*0101 (corresponding to the serological determinants DR3 and DR52) – DQA1*0501-DQB1*0201 haplotype (52% vs. 19% of controls) and a strong secondary association with the DRB1*0401 allele (corresponding to the serological determinant DR4) (54% of DRB3*0101-negative patients compared with 23% of DRB3*0101-negative controls). In addition, molecular genotyping studies failed to demonstrate significant associations with either DQA, DQB or DPB other than those expected by linkage with DRB[1,2]. A weak association at the HLA DPB locus was also found, suggesting that the DRB region is the primary HLA Class II susceptibility region in AIH. Whether there is a common susceptibility determinant shared by DRB1*0301, DRB3*0101 and DRB1*0401, and which of the two DRB alleles is the primary susceptibility (or severity) allele in Caucasians remain unanswered questions.

There does appear to be a common susceptibility determinant carried by both the DRB1*0301 and DRB3*0101 alleles and the DRB1*0401 allele. A detailed analysis of the amino acid sequences encoded by these susceptibility alleles revealed a particular motif Leu-Leu-Glu-Gln-Lys-Arg (single letter code LLEQKR) at positions 67–72 of the DRBβ polypeptide, which is encoded by DRB1*0301, DRB3*0101 and DRB1*0401. The critical amino acid in this motif may be the lysine residue at position 71 of the HLA DRβ polypeptide. This motif was found in 94% of Caucasian patients studied compared with 64% of control subjects. In the Japanese, however, where the predominant DR4 allele in the DR4 serotype AIH patients has been found to be DRB1*0405, this does not appear to be the case. Those patients lacking DRB1*04 were all DR2-positive. Neither of these alleles encodes a lysine residue at position 71, although the DRB1*0405 allele encodes LLEQ at position 67–70 with arginine at position 72 and at the critical position 71.

In contrast to the findings in the Japanese, recent unpublished data suggest that the most common northern European DR2 allele (DRB1*1501) may actually be associated with resistance to AIH. It is of interest that this allele also encodes an arginine at position 71. To encompass these discordant observations, a second hypothesis suggests that the basic amino acids at position 13 of the DRβ-polypeptide encoded by all the DRB1*04 and DR2 alleles are responsible for AIH susceptibility in the Japanese. In children, HLA DR3 is increased in type 1 but not type 2 disease and HLA DR4 is decreased in both, suggesting DR4 may confer protection in the paediatric age group.

In early HLA studies in PBC, no Class I association was found, nor was there a consensus about an association with an HLA DR serotype. Currently, there is a consensus that there is a real, albeit weak association with DR8 in both Europe and the USA and a much stronger association in Japan where DR8 is more common in the general population. Although the data from Europe and the USA suggest that the association with the DRB1*0801 allele is stronger than for either DQA, DQB or DPB, there is controversy over whether DRB1*0803 or the linked DPB1*0501 allele is the primary susceptibility allele in Japanese patients.

Early serological investigations of HLA in PSC demonstrated associations with HLA B8 and DR3, and a secondary association with DR2. More recently, PCR genotyping has addressed the validity of the serotype associations in PSC. One survey of the distribution of HLA Class II DR, DQA and DQB alleles in PSC was undertaken by Farrant *et al.* of the King's College group in the UK[3]. The HLA DRB1*0301-DRB3*0101-DQA1*0501-DQB1*0201 haplotype was found in 39% of patients compared with 19% of controls. This study, however, could not confirm the secondary association with a DR2 serotype. The association with DRB1*0301 in this study was weak and only strongly significant as part of the A1-B8-DRB1*0301-DRB3*0101 haplotype. A new association with the DRB1*1301-DRB3*0101-DQA1*0103-DQB1*0603 haplotype and a negative association with the DRB1*0401 allele were also described in Farrant's study. The association with DRB1*1301 partly explains the lower frequency of DRB1*0301 in this study compared with the earlier data which were based on serology where antigens belonging to cross-reactive groups may have been misclassified.

Following Farrant's publication, the Oxford group[4] also showed that susceptibility to PSC is determined by HLA DRB1*0301 and DRB3*0101; a Swedish study[5] found associations with the DRB1*0301, DRB3*0101 alleles and with the DRB1*1301-DQA1*0102-DQB1*0603 haplotype. There is, however, considerable controversy over the interpretation of the data from these three studies. In Farrant's analysis, it was suggested that DRB3*0101 may be the primary susceptibility allele as DRB3*0101 is present on both susceptibility haplotypes (i.e. those containing DRB1*0301 and DRB1*1301) and accounts for 55% of patients compared with 44% for DRB1*0301 and 24% for DRB1*1301. Further analysis suggested that there is a weak secondary association with the DR2 haplotype DRB1*1501-DRB5*0101 in DR3-negative patients. Overall, DRB3*0101 and DRB5*0101 were present in 79% of patients in Farrant's series. Since these two DRB alleles encode a leucine residue at position 38 of the DRBβ polypeptide, while all other DRB alleles encode alanine or valine at position 38, a model of susceptibility based on leucine at position 38 was proposed. Although the Oxford group agreed that DRB3*0101 is the primary susceptibility allele in PSC, and with the leucine at position 38 hypothesis, this was not the interpretation of the Swedish group, who argued instead that the association of PSC with DRB3*0101 is simply the result of linkage disequilibrium. Since there is very little difference in the results of these three studies, it is not possible to judge them on the basis of the raw data or statistics of each individual study. By pooling the data, a clear association with DRB3*0101 is found which is much stronger than that with DRB1*0301. Since data on DRB1*1301 are only available for two out of the three studies, it is not possible to consider DRB1*1301 vs. DRB3*0101.

The original idea that DR4 may be protective in PSC was refuted by studies from Oxford and Sweden, although pooled data and analysis of more recent unpublished data point to a negative association with DR4 which is not simply due to the over-representation of DRB1*0301 and DRB3*0101. DR4 does not appear to be associated with a poor prognosis in PSC as was suggested in the Oxford data.

HLA-ASSOCIATIONS OF INFLAMMATORY BOWEL DISEASE

Genetic studies of inflammatory bowel disease (ulcerative colitis and Crohn's disease) have been directed at populations, families and twins, using a variety of measurements. Interpretation of results and comparisons among studies are difficult, however, not only because of ethnic variations, but because of the heterogeneity of inflammatory bowel disease *per se*. The division of inflammatory bowel disease into ulcerative colitis and Crohn's disease is a first major division of this entity, and even then some overlap occurs. In individual patients a clear distinction of the clinical phenotype may not be obvious and there are families in which cases of ulcerative colitis and Crohn's disease both occur. Within ulcerative colitis and Crohn's disease, many divisions are possible based on location, severity and various clinical features, such as the presence of extraintestinal manifestations, age of onset, presence of circulating antibodies, etc. Despite the presence of overlap in families in which ulcerative colitis and Crohn's disease both occur, family studies indicate that the two entities do not co-exist in the majority of familial inflammatory bowel disease. HLA studies have in general legitimized the division into the two major categories of ulcerative colitis and Crohn's disease.

Early serotyping studies of HLA Class I antigens and immunoglobulin heavy chain and light chain immunoglobulin allotypes demonstrated no convincing evidence of associations and/or linkages between postulated inflammatory bowel disease susceptibility loci and genes coding for HLA antigens or immunoglobulin allotypes[6]. More recent studies of serotyping or genotyping for HLA Class II genes have revealed some conflicting results, due in part to ethnic diversity.

Ulcerative colitis in Japanese populations is associated with HLA DR2[7]. Moreover, severe disease has been reported to be associated with the HLA DRB1*1502 allele with milder disease with the HLA DRB1*1501 allele. There appears to be a strong association of ulcerative colitis with glycine at position 86 of the DRBβ polypeptide[8]. Conflicting data exist for association of ulcerative colitis with DRB1 alleles in studies from the United Kingdom and North America. One study has uncovered an association with HLA DR2, but it was confined to pANCA-positive patients. A more recent investigation by Duerr and Neigut[9] found no association with HLA DR2 in pANCA-positive or -negative subgroups, but found a negative association with the HLA DRB1*1601 allele. An unpublished study from the USA has discovered an association of ulcerative colitis with HLA DR6. Of particular interest, vis-à-vis the discussion above regarding HLA associations in AIH and PSC, a study from France found that the haplotype HLA DRB1*0301-DQB1*0201 has a protective effect for ulcerative colitis (and Crohn's disease).

Crohn's disease appears to be associated with an HLA DR1-DQ5 haplotype. An even stronger association has been demonstrated in the MHC for tumour necrosis factor alleles which may represent an extension of the HLA haplotype. The DRB3*0101 allele was negatively associated with Crohn's disease in a recent North American study. In a Japanese population, a positive association with the HLA DQB1*04 allele and a negative association with the DQA1*0102 allele was reported.

It should be noted, however, that more data are accumulating which suggest that disease susceptibility loci independent of the MHC may exist for inflammatory bowel disease. Candidates include loci on chromosome 2 involving the IL-1 gene family for ulcerative colitis and loci on chromosome 16 which are likely to be involved in susceptibility to Crohn's disease[10]. This does not exclude the HLA loci on the short arm of chromosome 6 as being important, however, as several genetic loci are likely to be responsible for susceptibility to multifaceted diseases such as ulcerative colitis and Crohn's disease.

PRIMARY SCLEROSING CHOLANGITIS AND ULCERATIVE COLITIS

In addressing the patient with PSC and ulcerative colitis as the prototypical patient with autoimmune liver disease and an extrahepatic manifestation, and then applying the markers of pANCA and an HLA phenotype as surrogate markers of disease susceptibility (or severity), we face published data that are at times conflicting and/or confusing. For example, HLA alleles that seem to confer susceptibility to PSC seem to be associated with resistance to ulcerative colitis. It would seem logical to assume that other genes at other loci are important in determining disease occurrence or severity. Moreover, if we assume that the HLA gene products are truly involved in the immunopathogenesis of these disorders, rather than these genes being implicated by linkage or molecular mimicry, then it would be logical to study other members of the immunoglobulin supergene family as modulators of disease occurrence or severity. And since the crucial location for initiation of the ongoing necroinflammatory process in the liver and colon presumably is the HLA–peptide–TCR ternary complex, it would be logical also to study the TCR genes in patients with co-existing diseases. (Preliminary studies using restriction fragment polymorphism patterns in patients with inflammatory bowel disease without co-existing autoimmune liver disease did not reveal any association with inherited TCRα or β alleles.)

We propose, therefore, that a study of both HLA and TCR genotypes in patients with co-existing PSC and ulcerative colitis, stratified for pANCA positivity would be informative in defining the nature of genetic susceptibility and severity. Moreover, such studies in multiplex families of patients in which both disorders exist, providing relative homogeneity to the study population, would permit segregation analysis to identify true linkage between any disease susceptibility loci and the polymorphic members of the immunoglobulin supergene family. This may identify multiple inheritance patterns. As methods for defining TCR genes improve, it may also become possible to identify TCR gene repertoires associated with HLA inheritance and/or disease status. It may be that TCR repertoire bias provides the pathway through which HLA modulates disease occurrence and/or severity. Such studies may therefore reveal some of the genetic mechanisms which determine the extrahepatic manifestations of autoimmune liver disease.

References

1. Manabe K, Donaldson PT, Underhill JA et al. HLA A1-B8-DR3-DQ2-DPB1*0401 extended haplotype in autoimmune hepatitis. Hepatology. 1993;18:1334–7.
2. Donaldson PT, Doherty DG, Hayllar KM, McFarlane I, Johnson PJ, Williams R. Susceptibility to autoimmune chronic active hepatitis: Human leucocyte antigens DR4 and A1-B8-DR3 are independent risk factors. Hepatology. 1991;13:701–6.
3. Farrant JM, Doherty DG, Donaldson PT et al. Amino acid substitutions at position 38 of the DRβ polypeptide confer susceptibility and protection from primary sclerosing cholangitis. Hepatology. 1992;16:390–5.
4. Mehal WZ, Lo Y-MD, Wordsworth BP et al. HLA DR4 is a marker for rapid disease progression in primary sclerosing cholangitis. Gastroenterology. 1994;106:160–7.
5. Olerup O, Olsson R, Hultcrantz R, Broome U. HLA-DR and HLA-DQ are not markers for rapid disease progression in primary sclerosing cholangitis. Gastroenterology. 1995;108:870–8.
6. Gudjonsson H, Schanfield MS, Albertini RJ, McAuliffe TL, Beeken WL, Krawitt EL. Association and linkage studies of immunoglobulin heavy chain allotypes in inflammatory bowel disease. Tissue Antigens. 1988;31:243–9.
7. Toyoda H, Wang S-J, Yang H-Y et al. Distinct associations of HLA Class II genes with inflammatory bowel disease. Gastroenterology. 1993;104:741–8.
8. Futami S, Aoyama N, Honsako Y et al. HLA-DRB1*1502 allele, subtype of DR15, is associated with susceptibility to ulcerative colitis and its progression. Dig Dis Sci. 1995;40:814–18.
9. Duerr RH, Neigut DA. Molecularly defined HLA-DR2 alleles in ulcerative colitis and an anti-neutrophil cytoplasmic antibody-positive subgroup. Gastroenterology. 1995;108:423–7.
10. Hugot J-P, Laurent-Pulg P, Gower-Rousseau C et al. Mapping of a susceptibility locus for Crohn's disease on chromosome 16. Nature. 1996;379:821–3.

7
Immunological and clinical aspects of autoimmune hepatitis

K.-H. MEYER ZUM BÜSCHENFELDE

DEFINITION AND CHARACTERISTICS OF AUTOIMMUNE HEPATITIS

Acute and chronic inflammatory liver diseases resulting from autoimmunity are distinct entities in which immune reactions against host antigens are believed to be a major pathogenetic mechanism (Table 1)[1]. Increasing evidence for this has been accumulated, particularly in autoimmune hepatitis (AIH), a disease with characteristics first described by Waldenström in 1950[2] and Kunkel et al. in 1951[3]. Today AIH, like other autoimmune disorders, is regarded as a clinical syndrome occurring in both sexes and all age groups with a marked female predominance and frequent associations with other autoimmune disorders. Most patients present with typical clinical manifestations. Hepatomegaly and splenomegaly are the most common abnormal physical findings. The abnormalities of the immune system include polyclonal hyper-γ-globulinaemia, autoantibodies as diagnostic markers, genetic associations with HLA-A1, B8, DR3 or DR4 and an increased CD4/CD8 ratio in peripheral blood and liver tissue. Epidemiological and virological studies suggest that AIH cannot be attributed to the presence of hepatic viruses A–G or to metabolic and drug-induced liver diseases (Table 2)[4–9].

Clinical, biochemical and histological features and the specificity of circulating autoantibodies were used in the development of diagnostic criteria by a panel of experts (the International Autoimmune Hepatitis Group)[10] during the meeting of the International Association For The Study Of The Liver in Brighton, UK, 1992 (Table 3). Although the panel voted against the subdivision of AIH based on marker

Table 1. Classification of autoimmune liver disease

Cholestatic		*Hepatic*
Primary biliary cirrhosis		Autoimmune hepatitis types I, II, III
Primary sclerosing cholangitis		
	Autoimmune cholangitis	
	Overlap syndromes	

Table 2. Characteristics of AIH

- Inflammatory hepatocellular disease
- Natural course
  - Long subclinical with slow elevating liver function test followed by a fluctuating disease activity prior to diagnosis
  - Up to 40% present with an acute hepatitis
  - Frequently cirrhosis at the time of diagnosis
- Cryptogenic nature (not attributed to viral, drug or metabolic LD)
- Female predominance (>80%)
- Hepatosplenomegaly most common physical finding
- Frequently associated with other autoimmune disorders
- Polyclonal hyper-γ-globulinaemia
- High incidence of serum autoantibodies
- Association with HLA Class I and II
- Increased CD4/CD8 ratio in peripheral blood and liver infiltrating lymphocytes
- Rapid and complete response to immunosuppression

Table 3. Definition of autoimmune hepatitis

Parameters	*Score*
• Hyper-γ-globulinaemia	+3
• Autoantibodies:	
ANA, SMA, LKM1	+3
SLA, ASGPR, LC, LP, HHPM	+2
AMA	−2
• Female sex (80–90%)	+2
• Benefit from immunosuppression	+2
• Genetics: B8-DR3 or DR4	+1
• HBsAg, IgM anti-HAV	−3

From the International Autoimmune Hepatitis Group, 1992, Reference 10

autoantibodies, a subgrouping of AIH is reasonable and justified by differences in patient populations, some clinical features and prognosis.

AIH type I, characterized by antinuclear antibodies (ANA) and smooth muscle antibodies (SMA) is the most common type of AIH accounting for about 60–70% of patients. Low titres of antimitochondrial antibodies (AMA) are found in about 20% of this group without biliary changes when they are investigated by histopathology or cholangiography, but biliary lesions which are typical for primary biliary cirrhosis (PBC) and primary sclerosing cholangitis (PSC) with positive tests for ANA or SMA should not be regarded as criteria for the diagnosis of AIH, even when there is a good response to immunosuppression.

AIH type II is characterized by autoantibodies against microsomal antigens of liver and kidney (LKM1)[11] in the absence of ANA and SMA. AIH type II is a rare disease accounting for only 5% of patients with AIH. About 70% of the patients have an onset at a young age, between two and fourteen years, and about half of the patients have an association with other immune disorders. Most patients present with acute onset, severe course and quick progression to liver failure or cirrhosis of the liver.

AIH type III represents a poorly defined group of AIH patients (Table 4). Only 70% of patients with AIH have one of the classic autoantibody markers, such as ANA or SMA (type I AIH) or (LM1 type II AIH). Tests for autoantibodies to

Table 4. AIH type III

- Not well-defined group of AIH
- About 30–40% of patients with AIH
- Common findings:
  - Hyper-γ-globulinaemia and selective IgG elevation
  - No attribution to hepatitis viruses A–E
  - Positive for HLA A1, B8, DR3 or DR4
- Confirmation of diagnosis:
  - marker auto ABs against SLA, LC1, LP and/or ASGPR

  or if negative:
  - Differential therapy with immunosuppressive drugs

soluble liver antigen (SLA)[12], liver cytosolic antigen (LC1)[13], antigen of liver and pancreas (LP)[14], the asialoglycoprotein receptor (ASGPR)[15,16] and some other so-far poorly characterized autoantigens of the hepatocellular plasma membrane[1,17–19] can help to identify AIH in most cases, especially in patients with hyper-γ-globulinaemia, selective increase of serum IgG levels and a typical HLA-pattern. Unfortunately, assays for these autoantibodies are restricted to a very few laboratories. It is therefore important to note that the absence of autoantibodies at presentation should not exclude the diagnosis of AIH. This holds true for about 30% of patients whose diagnosis may be missed because of incomplete autoantibody testing. Application of the entire panel of autoantibodies reduces the number of autoantibody-negative AIH patients to less than 5–10% in our experience. If in these remaining patients, the clinical findings are still suggestive but not definitive, a prompt complete response to immunosuppressive drugs may help to confirm the diagnosis[9,45].

LIVER MEMBRANE AUTOANTIGENS AS TARGETS IN AIH

Marker-autoantibodies are the hallmark of autoimmune liver diseases. However, their target antigens are mainly located intracellularly and lack organ specificity. This fact makes it difficult to understand their origin and immune pathogenetic role. We therefore began, as long ago as the 1960s[20], investigations to identify autoantigens expressed on the plasma membrane of hepatocytes. At that time, a crude plasma membrane preparation with organ-specific components, later named liver specific protein (LSP)[21], received clinical and experimental attention. It was possible to induce an autoimmune liver disease in animal models[22,23] and to detect T cell reactivity and autoantibodies to LSP and its components[24–26] in AIH but to a lesser extent in other inflammatory liver diseases, particularly in PBC. In follow-up studies, anti-LSP autoantibodies could be used to predict the clinical outcome of AIH in men and had clinical relevance[27]. The further search for the relevant target antigens in LSP preparations led to the detection and characterization of autoantigens as part of LSP. As components of LSP, the human asialoglycoprotein receptor (hASGPR)[28], a 43-kDa protein[29], a 26-kDa liver membrane antigen (LMA)[18] and a partially liver-specific 60-kDa membrane antigen[30] have been identified by autoantibodies and monoclonal antibodies. Whereas autoantibodies to the hASGPR had clinical relevance[15,16], further studies are needed to characterize the autoepitopes of the other above-mentioned membrane antigens.

Table 5. Liver membrane antigens as targets in AIH

LSP
• Induction of AIH-like disease in animal models (rabbits 1968, 1972 and mice 1990)
• T-cell reactivity to LSP and its components
• Auto ABs against LSP
LSP-related autoantigens
• ASGPR (T and B cell epitopes)
• 43-kDa protein (liver specific, identified by MAB)
• 26-kDa protein (identified by auto ABs)
• 60-kDa protein (identified by auto ABs, partially liver specific)
• Further proteins of small MW fractions
Membrane-expressed cytosolic antigens
• Liver–kidney microsomal antigen (LKM1)

Little is known about the physiological expression of cytosolic antigens on the surface of hepatocytes. In the case of LKM_1 antigens, membrane expression has been studied intensively. So far, the amount remains questionable and it may only exist at a very low level[31], but the description of liver-infiltrating autoreactive CD4+ LKM_1-specific T-cell responses in LKM_1-antibody-positive AIH and the correlation of this immune response with disease activity support a pathogenetic significance of LKM autoantigens as targets in AIH (Table 5)[32,33,45].

T-CELL AUTOREACTIVITY TO LIVER MEMBRANE AUTOANTIGENS

Studies of cell-mediated immunity against LSP were extended to the ASGPR in the 1980s[34]. Circulating T lymphocytes that were sensitized against the human ASGPR in patients with AIH were described. All patients showing this type of T-cell reactivity had signs of active disease at the time of the study. In addition, T-cell clones from liver biopsies taken from patients with AIH were established. Approximately 10% of these clones responded specifically to human ASGPR. The response was restricted to autologous antigen-presenting cells and HLA Class II recognition. The majority of the T-cell clones exhibited the CD4-positive CD8-negative phenotype[35]. The T cells were able to stimulate B cells in an antigen-specific manner to produce autoantibodies against the human ASGPR[36]. Studies with low-molecular-weight soluble liver antigens obtained from LSP preparations in patients with AIH provide support for further T-cell-target antigens and T-cell autoreactivity in the majority of our AIH patients, but not in patients with PBC or other liver diseases or autoimmune disorders[25] (Figure 1). The reactivity was almost exclusively confined to patients with active and progressive disease. The recovery of AIH was associated with an antigen-specific and an antigen-non-specific T-cell suppression suggesting a generalized spontaneous immunosuppression that may be more pronounced *in vivo* than can be measured *in vitro* (Figure 2).

It has been demonstrated that liver-infiltrating T-cell clones from patients with type II AIH recognize a recombinant LKM_1 antigen carrying the immunodominant 33-amino-acid regions of cytochrome P_{450} II D6, the main target of LKM_1 autoantibodies[32]. The analysis of the fine specificity of the cellular immune response

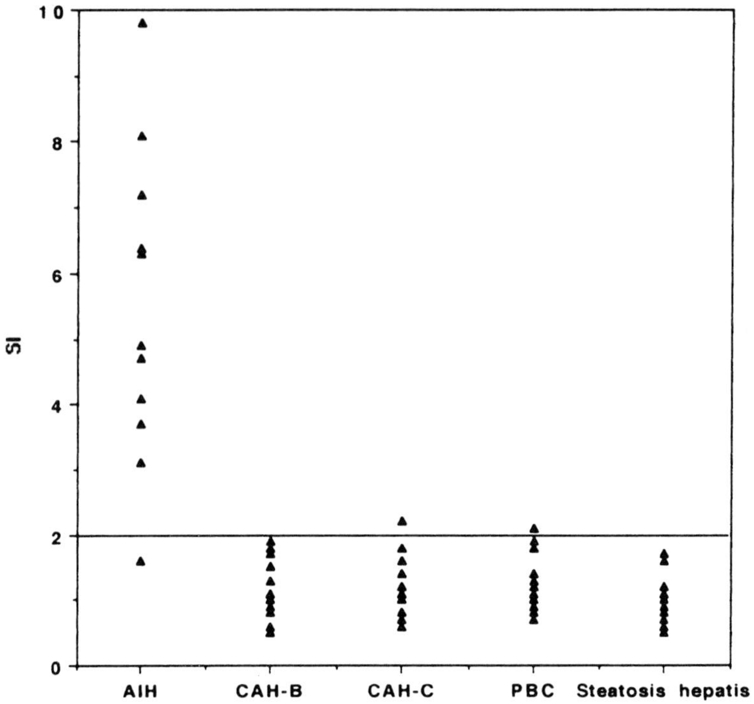

Figure 1. Proliferative responses of peripheral blood leukocytes from patients with autoimmune hepatitis (AIH), chronic viral hepatitis B (CAH-B), chronic viral hepatitis C (CAH-C), primary biliary cirrhosis (PBC) or fatty liver (steatosis hepatis) to soluble human liver antigens (small molecular weight fraction of 100000*g* supernatant of liver homogenate). The results are given as stimulation indices (cpm in wells containing antigen divided by cpm in wells containing no antigen), with a stimulation index of more than 2 considered to constitute a positive response

to the main T-cell epitopes within the immunodominant LKM_1 antigen showed that CD4+ T-cell isolated and expanded from blood and liver tissue of AIH patients react in a HLA Class II-restricted manner and secrete large amounts of IFNγ. A major T-cell epitope in AIH was identified that was recognized by TH1 helper cells. Furthermore, it has been shown that PBMC recognize autologous LKM_1-specific T cells, suggesting the presence of a regulatory T-cell network in the control of autoreactive T cells as well as T cells responsive to the activation state. Interestingly, the LKM-specific T-cell response was detectable in all patients with AIH type II but also in 6 of 12 patients with AIH type I and in 4 of 31 patients with chronic hepatitis C (Table 6; Figure 3)[33].

These observations contribute to our understanding of the natural course of AIH, indicating that AIH could be the result of a long-lasting battle between autoreactive effector cells and their at-times insufficient down-regulating counterparts. Keeping in mind the models of T-cell-mediated liver injury in mice, it is most likely that the induction of a pathogenetic T-cell response is the consequence of a locally activated immune system and a destroyed physiological interplay between hepatocytes and non-parenchymal liver cells by cytokines. Further

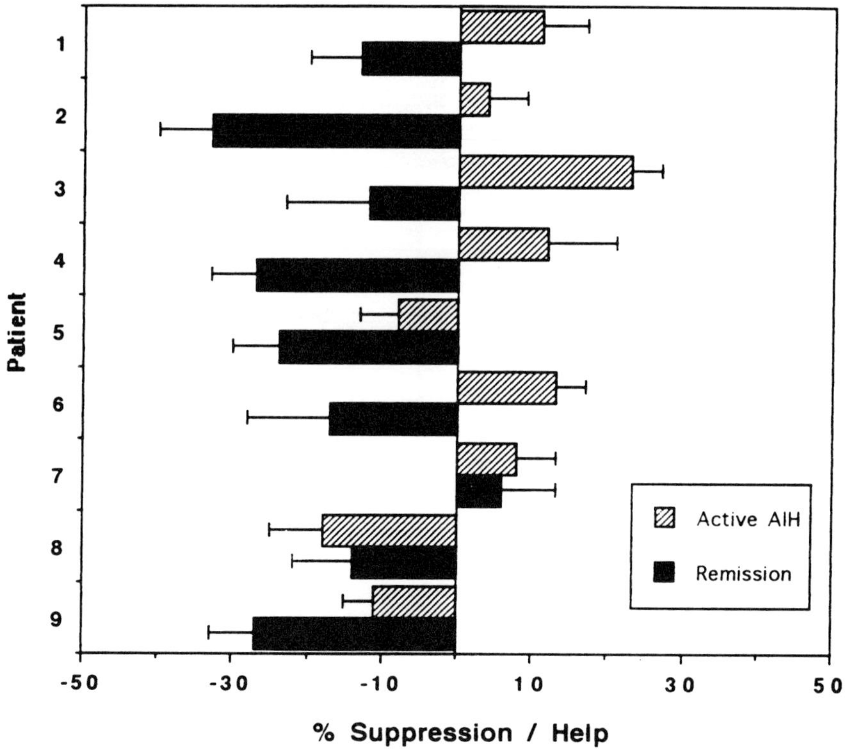

Figure 2. Helper/suppressor activity of peripheral blood leukocytes (PBL) from 9 patients with autoimmune hepatitis (AIH) measured during active disease and in remission. Results are expressed as % change. Irradiated PBL from the two disease phases were added to PBL from the acute disease phase that were stimulated with human soluble liver antigen fractions. Positive values mean an increase in cpm by adding irradiated PBL, and thus help; negative values mean a decrease, and therefore suppression

Table 6. Autoreactive CD4+ LKM-specific T-cell response in AIH

	n	*Anti-LKM1 AB*		*LKM T-cell reactivity*	
		+	−	+	%
AIH type I	12	0	12	6	50
AIH type II	8	8	0	8	100
Chronic HC	31	2	29	4	12.9

studies are needed to analyse the CD4-positive T-cell subpopulations involved. TH1 cells have a higher cytotoxic capacity than TH2 cells and secrete cytokines that can affect the synthesis, function and structure of the above-mentioned liver-membrane and cytosolic antigens[37]. The role of non-parenchymal liver cells and the genetically determined factors responsible for susceptibility and resistance require more detailed study.

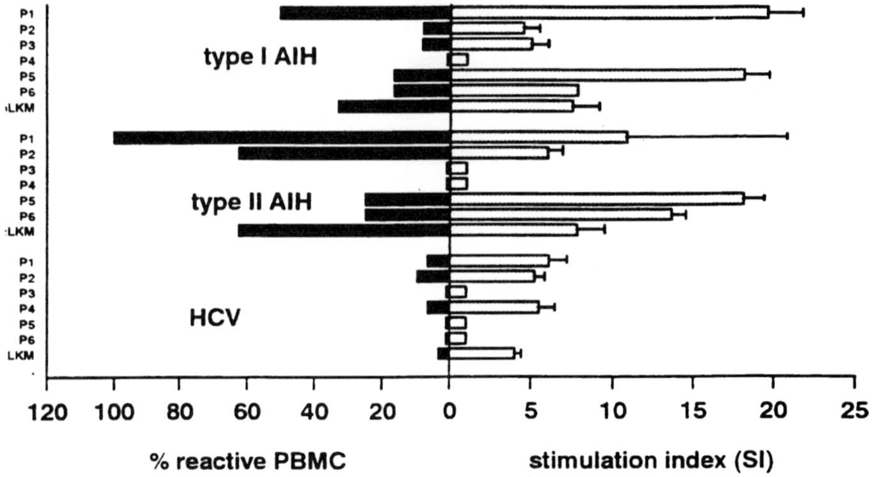

Figure 3. Autoreactive CD4+ LKM-specific T-cell response in AIH. Relative frequencies of patients with type I or II AIH or chronic hepatitis C that showed a proliferative PBMC response to LKM peptides P1–6 or the crude microsomal protein fraction (nLKM). Mean stimulation index (SI) ± standard deviations

AUTOANTIBODIES AGAINST LIVER MEMBRANE ANTIGENS

Keeping in mind the monophasic course of experimental AIH in mice, it is clear that there must be additional factors causing this chronic fluctuating and self-perpetuating disease. There is now increasing evidence that, in the chronic phase of the disease, liver membrane autoantibodies are involved. The first hint of this was the *in-vivo* binding of IgG in a linear pattern to the surface of isolated hepatocytes taken from liver biopsies in AIH[38,39]. The essential role of the humoral autoimmune response in AIH received further support from experimental models in rabbits[38]. A monoclonal antibody against a 43-kDa liver surface antigen was able to induce acute liver injury and lysis of hepatocytes *in vivo* and *in vitro*[29]. In the absence of serum or T-cell components of the immune system, it is likely that *in vivo* the monoclonal antibodies cooperate with K cells via ADCC. Additional information from liver perfusion studies using anti-ASGPR antibodies has shown that anti-ASGPR antibodies bind or are consumed predominantly in the periportal zone of the hepatic lobule[40]. Since periportal inflammatory infiltrates predominate and are a characteristic of AIH, ADCC may be responsible in part for the destruction of periportal hepatocytes. This notion is further supported by *in-vitro* studies showing that non-T-cell lymphocytes (K cells from the peripheral blood) have cytotoxic activity to autologous hepatocytes isolated from liver biopsies in AIH. Again it is likely that K cells may be responsible for liver cell lysis via *in-vivo* autoantibodies bound to the surface of hepatocytes[1] (Table 7).

Among the established liver membrane-related autoantigens, the ASGPR represents to date the component of the hepatic plasma membrane which is fully characterized. Assays for the detection of anti-ASGPR are reliable. The clinical

Table 7. Mechanisms of liver injury in AIH – Role of liver-membrane auto-ABs

- *In-vitro* binding of IgG to hepatocytes in human and animal disease
- Acute liver injury and lyses of hepatocytes *in vivo* and *in vitro* by a MAB against a 43-kDa membrane antigen
- Consumption of anti-ASGPR in the periportal zone of the hepatic lobule
- ADCC to autologous hepatocytes *in vitro*
- Correlation between anti-LSP and -ASGPR to disease activity and their disappearance under immunosuppression

Table 8. Autoepitopes on human ASGPR

Epitope	*Definition*	*Detection*
Conformational	Exclusively detected on native ASGPR-heteromers	Enzyme immunoassay
Peptide-specific	Detected on cyanogen-bromide fragments or tryptic fragments of ASGPR	Immunoblot or enzyme immunoassay
Glycosides	Abolished after deglycosylation of ASGPR	Immunoblot or enzyme immunoassay
Ligand-binding domain	Inhibition of ligand binding	*In vitro* uptake of asialofetuin

data support the utility of measuring anti-ASGPR during differential diagnosis of patients with chronic inflammatory liver disease (prevalence >80% in AIH of all subtypes) and during their follow-up (down-regulation or elimination during response to immunosuppressive therapy)[16,41]. Furthermore, four immunodominant epitopes for anti-ASGPR have been identified (Table 8). Anti-ASGPR autoantibodies reacting particularly with glycoside but also with ligand-binding domain epitopes have been detected selectively in patients with AIH and seem to be highly disease specific. The role of so-far characterized ASGPR epitopes for the pathogenesis of AIH has to be clarified in future studies (unpublished data, Dr Treichel), but the close correlation of anti-ASGPR autoantibodies to disease activity and their disappearance under immunosuppression further support the pathogenetic role *in vivo*. In contrast, antinuclear antibodies and some anticytosolic autoantibodies are detectable in patients with AIH after months and years in remission.

CONCLUDING REMARKS

Initially, many patients with AIH run a long subclinical course with only slowly elevating liver function test followed by a fluctuating disease activity prior to diagnosis. Up to 40% of cases present with acute, sometimes fulminant, hepatitis. The early clinical observation that many patients with AIH already have cirrhosis of the liver at the time of diagnosis is still true today. The main reasons for this are that diagnosis is still made too late in a considerable number of patients but, more importantly, about one third of patients with AIH remain undiagnosed because of incomplete autoantibody testing, a problem that must be solved in the near future.

Most autoimmune disorders involve a genetic background[5,30,42,43]. This is also true for AIH. Different environmental factors are frequently able to induce transient autoimmune phenomena but not autoimmune disease as distinct from a disease promoting genetically determined background for autoimmunity. It has been shown by several investigators that autoimmune reactions against membrane antigens of hepatocytes can be induced by all hepatitis viruses and some non-hepatic viruses or their cytokines released during viral infection, but do not usually run to self-perpetuating autoimmune liver disease[6]. Only very few case reports of AIH following acute hepatitis A or B have been published so far[44]. As different environmental factors alone are not sufficient to trigger a self-perpetuating autoimmune response, a transformation of the naturally occurring non-pathogenetic autoimmune response into a pathological autoreactivity must be considered as a further important prerequisite for the induction and perpetuation of autoimmune liver injury[25]. The natural course of AIH is in agreement with this notion and is likely to be the expression of a relevant imbalance between autoreactive and counter-regulatory forces. The experimental models of AIH have shown that the initial phase of AIH is characterized by the presence of a liver membrane autoantigen-reactive CD4-positive T cell in the peripheral blood. Their role in the initiation and pathogenesis of human AIH requires more detailed studies. In the later self-perpetuating phase of human AIH, an autoantibody-mediated liver injury may be an important or even the dominating pathogenetic factor. This is particularly based on the close correlation between disease activity and liver- and disease-specific circulating or rather *in-vivo* liver membrane-bound autoantibodies[45].

References

1. Meyer zum Büschenfelde K-H, Lohse AW, Manns M, Poralla T. Autoimmunity and liver disease. Hepatology. 1990;12:354–63.
2. Waldström J. Leber, Blutproteine und Nahrungseiweiss. 8. Tagung Stoffwechsel-Krh., Bad Kissingen, Sonderband XV. 1950:113–19.
3. Kunkel HG, Ahrens JR, Eisenmenger WJ, Bongiovanni AM, Slater RJ. Extreme hypergammaglobulinemia in young women with liver disease of unknown etiology. J Clin Invest. 1951;30:654.
4. Aiza I, Chiff ER. Autoimmune hepatitis. Curr Opin Gastroenterol. 1995;11:238–44.
5. Czaja AJ, Carpenter HA, Santrach PJ, Moore SB. Genetic predispositions for the immunological features of chronic active hepatitis. Hepatology. 1993;18:816–22
6. Lohse AW, Gerken G, Mohr H et al. Relation between autoimmune liver diseases and viral hepatitis: clinical and serological characteristics in 859 patients. Ger J Gastroenterol. 1995;33:527–33.
7. Mackay IR, Morris PJ. Association of autoimmune chronic active hepatitis with HLA-A1, A2, B8. Lancet. 1972;2:793–5.
8. Mackay IR, Taft LI, Cowling DC. Lupoid hepatitis. Lancet. 1956;2:1323–6.
9. Meyer zum Büschenfelde K-H, Lohse AW. Autoimmune hepatitis. N Engl J Med. 1995;333: 1084–5.
10. Johnsohn PJ, McFarlane IG. Meeting report: International Autoimmune Hepatitis Group. Hepatology. 1993;18:998–1005.
11. Manns M, Johnson EF, Griffen KJ, Tan EM, Sullivan KF. Major antigen of liver kidney microsomal autoantibodies in idiopathic autoimmune hepatitis is cytochrome P450 db. J Clin Invest. 1989;83: 1066–72.
12. Manns M, Gerken G, Kyriatsoules A, Staritz M, Meyer zum Büschenfelde K-H. Characterization of a new subgroup of autoimmune chronic active hepatitis by autoantibodies against a soluble liver antigen. Lancet. 1987;1:292–4.

13. Martini E, Nisen A, Cavalli F et al. Antibodies to liver cytosol (Anti-LC_1) in patients with autoimmune chronic active hepatitis. Hepatology. 1988;8:1662–6.
14. Berg PA, Stechemesser E. Hypergammaglobulinämische chronisch aktive Hepatitis mit Nachweis komplementbindender partiell leberspezifischer Antikörper. Verh Dtsch Ges zum Med. 1981; 87:921.
15. McFarlane BM, McSorley CG, Vergani D, McFarlane IG, Williams R. Serum autoantibodies reacting with the hepatic asialoglycoprotein receptor protein (hepatic lectin) in acute and chronic liver disorders. J Hepatol. 1986;3:196–205.
16. Treichel U, McFarlane BM, Takeshi S et al. Demographics of anti-asialoglycoprotein receptor autoantibodies in autoimmune hepatitis. Gastroenterology. 1994;107:799–804.
17. Hopf U, Meyer zum Büschenfelde K-H, Arnold W. Detection of a liver membrane autoantibody in HBs-Ag-negative chronic hepatitis. N Engl J Med. 1976;294:578–82.
18. Hopf U, Jahn HU, Möller B et al. Liver membrane antibodies (LMA) recognize a 26-kD protein on the hepatocellular surface. Clin Exp Immunol. 1990;79:54–61.
19. Swanson NR, Reed WD, Yarred LJ, Shilkin KB, Joske RA. Autoantibodies to isolated plasma membranes in chronic active hepatitis. II. Specificity of antibodies. Hepatology. 1990;11:613–21.
20. Meyer zum Büschenfelde K-H, Schrank CH. Untersuchungen zur Frage organspezifischer Antigene der Leber. Klinische Woschenschrift. 1966;44:654–6.
21. Meyer zum Büschenfelde K-H, Miescher PA. Liver specific antigens, purification and characterization. Clin Exp Immunol. 1972;10:89–102.
22. Lohse A, Manns M, Dienes H-P, Meyer zum Büschenfelde K-H, Cohen IR. Experimental autoimmune hepatitis: disease induction, time course and T-cell reactivity. Hepatology. 1990;11:24–30.
23. Meyer zum Büschenfelde K-H, Kössling FK, Miescher PA. Experimental chronic active hepatitis in rabbits following immunization with human liver proteins. Clin Exp Immunol. 1972;10: 99–108.
24. Jensen DM, McFarlane IG, Portmann BS, Eddleston ALWF, Williams R. Detection of antibodies directed against liver-specific membrane lipoprotein in patients with acute and chronic active hepatitis. N Engl J Med. 1978;299:1–7.
25. Lohse AW, Kögel M, Meyer zum Büschenfelde K-H. Evidence for spontaneous immunosuppression in autoimmune hepatitis. Hepatology. 1995;22:381–8.
26. Manns M, Meyer zum Büschenfelde K-H, Hess G. Autoantibodies against liver specific protein: studies on disease-, species- and organ-specificity. Gut. 1980;21:955–61.
27. McFarlane IG, Hegarty JE, McSorley CG, McFarlane BM, Wiliams R. Antibodies to liver-specific protein predict outcome of treatment withdrawal in autoimmune chronic active hepatitis. Lancet. 1984;2:954–6.
28. McFarlane IG, McFarlane BM, Major GN, Tolley P, Williams R. Identification of the hepatic asialoglycoprotein receptor (hepatic lectin) as a component of liver specific membrane lipoprotein (LSP). Clin Exp Immunol. 1984;55:347–54.
29. Poralla T, Ramadori G, Dienes H-P et al. Liver cell damage caused by monoclonal antibody against an organ-specific membrane antigen in vivo and in vitro. J Hepatol. 1987;4:373–80.
30. Seki T, Kiyosawa K, Inoko H, Ota M. Association of auto-immune hepatitis with HLA-Bw 54 and DR4 in Japanese patients. Hepatology. 1990;12:1300–4.
31. Loeper J, Descatoire V, Maurice M et al. Presence of functional cytochrome P450 on isolated rat hepatocyte plasma membrane. Hepatology. 1990;11:145–53.
32. Löhr H, Manns M, Kyriatsoulis A et al. Clonal analysis of liver-infiltrating T cells in patients with LKM-1 antibody-positive autoimmune chronic active hepatitis. Clin Exp Immunol. 1991;84: 297–302.
33. Löhr H, Schlaak JF, Lohse AW et al. Autoreactive CD4+ LKM-specific and anticlonotypic T-cell responses in LKM-1 antibody-positive autoimmune hepatitis. Hepatology. 1996;24:6.
34. Wen L, Peakman M, Lobo-Yeo A et al. T-cell-directed hepatocyte damage in autoimmune chronic active hepatitis. Lancet. 1990;336:1527–30.
35. Löhr H, Treichel U, Poralla T, Manns M, Meyer zum Büschenfelde K-H, Fleischer B. The human hepatic asialoglycoprotein receptor is a target antigen for liver-infiltrating T cells in autoimmune chronic active hepatitis and primary biliary cirrhosis. Hepatology. 1990;12:1314–20.
36. Löhr H, Treichel U, Poralla T, Manns M, Meyer zum Büschenfelde K-H, Fleischer B. Liver-infiltrating T-helper cells in autoimmune chronic active hepatitis stimulate the production of autoantibodies against the human asialoglycoprotein receptor in vitro. Clin Exp Immunol. 1992;88: 45–9.

37. Löhr H, Schlaak JF, Gerken G, Fleischer B, Dienes H-P, Meyer zum Büschenfelde K-H. Phenotypical analysis and cytokine release of liver-infiltrating and peripheral blood T lymphocytes from patients with chronic hepatitis of different etiology. Liver. 1994;14:161–6.
38. Hopf U, Meyer zum Büschenfelde K-H. Studies on the pathogenesis of experimental chronic hepatitis in rabbits. II. Demonstration of immunoglobulin on isolated hepatocytes. Br J Exp Pathol. 1974;55:509–13.
39. Hopf U, Arnold W, Meyer zum Büschenfelde K-H et al. Studies on the pathogenesis of chronic inflammatory liver diseases. I. Membrane-fixed IgG on isolated hepatocytes from patients. Clin Exp Immunol. 1975;22:1–8.
40. McFarlane BM, Sipos J, Gove CD et al. Antibodies against the hepatic asialoglycoprotein receptor perfused in situ preferentially attach to periportal liver cells in the rat. Hepatology. 1990;11: 408–15.
41. Treichel U, Gerken G, Rossol S, Rotthauwe HW, Meyer zum Büschenfelde K-H, Poralla T. Autoantibodies against the human asialoglycoprotein receptor: effects of therapy in autoimmune and virus-induced chronic active hepatitis. J Hepatol. 1993;19:55–63.
42. Donaldson PT, Doherty DG, Underhill GA, Williams R. The molecular genetic of autoimmune liver disease. Hepatology. 1994;20:225–39.
43. Inoko H, Kiyosawa K. HLA class II molecules and autoimmune hepatitis susceptibility in Japanese patients. Gastroenterology. 1992;103:1041–7.
44. Huppertz HI, Treichel U, Gassel AM et al. Autoimmune hepatitis following hepatitis A virus infection. J Hepatol. 1995;23:204–8.
45. Meyer zum Büschenfelde K-H, Dienes HP. Autoimmune hepatitis: Definition – classification – histopathology – immunopathogenesis. Virchows Archiv. 1996;429:1–12.

8
PBC/PSC: Natural course and long-term outcome

K.P. MAIER

PRIMARY BILIARY CIRRHOSIS (PBC)

PBC is a chronic cholestatic inflammatory liver disease, most commonly seen in middle-aged women and strongly associated with antimitochondrial antibody (AMA).

The disease may progress to cirrhosis and, ultimately, death. On the other hand, very early cases suggestive of asymptomatic PBC have been detected, probably without detectable effect on the life span. Therefore, the natural history of PBC must be regarded as quite variable. In this situation, a number of prognostic indices have been developed to help in predicting the natural course and to aid in the timing of liver transplantation in the individual patient.

The very early ('preclinical') phase

The widespread use of automated biochemical screening has resulted in an increased number of patients being diagnosed as having PBC.

Only very few data are available on the long-term outcome of this group of patients, characterized by AMA-positivity, normal alkaline phosphatase and a liver histology diagnostic of, or at least compatible with, PBC in most cases[1,2]. In a ten-year follow-up study, 76% developed symptoms of PBC and 83% had liver function tests persistently showing cholestasis[2]. The median time from first positive AMA test to persistently elevated alkaline phosphatase activity was 5.6 (0.9–19) years. Five of the 29 patients died. However, no deaths were liver related! Thus, most of the patients with very early ('preclinical') AMA-positive PBC, finally progressed to typical PBC. However, disease progression seemed to be very slow. The median follow-up of the 24 surviving patients since the first positive AMA test to the last follow-up review was 17.8 (11.0–23.9) years[2].

The asymptomatic phase

Approximately 10–15% of PBC patients are asymptomatic at the time of diagnosis[3–5]. Laboratory tests reveal cholestasis, AMA are positive and, if done, liver histology is suggestive of or even diagnostic for PBC.

Initially, it was reported that the survival in these patients is similar to that in an age- and sex-matched control population[6,7]. However, a more recent study failed to substantiate this early finding: 89% of asymptomatic patients developed one or more symptoms and liver histology progressed to cirrhosis in 67% of precirrhotic patients when followed for a median of 7.6 years[8]. A 4-fold increase in mortality-rate compared with a control group, matched for age, sex and race was noticed ($p<0.001$). In the longest study[5] of 35 asymptomatic patients followed for 24 years (median), predicted survival from the time of diagnosis was twice as long for asymptomatic patients as for symptomatic patients (16 vs. 7.5 years, $p<0.0001$). Again, survival-time of the asymptomatic group was lower than predicted for matched controls ($p<0.001$). However, this difference became statistically significant only after 11 years of follow-up!

The five-year survival rate of the asymptomatic patients is about 90%[5,9,10]. In some patients, asymptomatic at the time of diagnosis, the onset of symptoms was accurately recorded. They developed symptomatic PBC a mean of 5.3 years after initial presentation[5]. Once symptomatic, their survival was similar to those presenting with symptoms at the time of diagnosis.

For unknown reasons, some patients remained symptom free during a long follow-up period. Compared with those who finally developed symptoms, their median survival time was significantly longer (16.7 vs. 12.6 years)[5]. This group, although small, obviously has an excellent prognosis.

The symptomatic phase

In PBC, hepatic mortality is associated with the appearance of symptoms. Of 212 patients presenting with symptomatic PBC, the mean predicted survival from the time of diagnosis was 7.5 years[5]. The duration of the symptomatic phase, however, varies greatly. This may be due also to the definition of symptoms, which can vary from one study to the next. Moreover, the prognostic value of some clinical manifestations of the disease may be classified differently.

The terminal phase

As the liver fails, serum bilirubin concentration rises steadily during the last 2 years of life. Therefore, the terminal phase is characterized by jaundice (bilirubin >10 mg/dl) with or without signs of portal hypertension. In this situation, patients may be candidates for liver transplantation.

The post-transplant phase

Orthotopic liver transplantation is the only therapeutic option for end-stage PBC. The reported 5-year post-transplantation survival is 70%[11]. Most deaths occur in

Table 1. PBC – bilirubin as a prognostic factor

Serum bilirubin (2 values, 6 months apart)	*Mean (range) survival (years)*
>2 mg/dl	4.1 (2.7–6.1)
>6 mg/dl	2.1 (1.6–2.7)
>10 mg/dl	1.4 (1.1–1.8)

From Reference 15

Table 2. Independent clinical variables predictive of survival in PBC

Yale	*Europe*	*Mayo*	*Oslo*	*Glasgow*	*Australia*
Age	Age	Age	Variceal bleeding	Age	Age
Bilirubin	Bilirubin	Bilirubin	Bilirubin	Bilirubin	Bilirubin
Hepatomegaly	Albumin	Albumin		Ascites	Albumin
Fibrosis/cirrhosis	Cirrhoses	Prothrombin time		Variceal bleeding	
	Cholestasis	Oedema		Fibrosis	
				Cholestasis	
				Mallory's bodies	

the first three months after transplantation. Half a year after OLT, the survival probability in transplanted patients was significantly better as predicted (Mayo model) if the patient had been treated conservatively. After one year, the survival curve is almost flat. Rehabilitation of the successfully transplanted patients is usually excellent.

Does PBC recur in the transplanted liver?

It is known that IgM elevation and AMA positivity persist after OLT. Biochemical tests are not very useful to evaluate PBC recurrence in the post-OLT situation. Liver morphology can be more reliable. Using strict morphological criteria, recurrence rates are very low, ranging from 0 to 8%[12–14].

Factors predictive of prognosis in PBC

Prognostication in the individual patient with PBC remains problematic. Asymptomatic patients without jaundice generally do well for a long time. Clinically, symptoms are associated with a doubtful prognosis.

Nearly 20 years ago, the paramount importance of serum bilirubin as a prognostic factor was demonstrated[15]. After two successive bilirubin values above 2 mg/dl obtained half a year apart, mean survival was 4.1 years; above 6 mg/dl, 2.1 years; and above 10 mg/dl, 1.4 years (Table 1). In all later studies, serum bilirubin was the most important marker both for short-term as well as for long-term prognosis.

More recent prognostic models are based on the Cox regression analysis. This model can be used to analyse the importance of several variables simultaneously. Several prognostic scores have been established (Table 2). Again, the only variable common to all models is the serum bilirubin level. Obviously, neither transaminases nor alkaline phosphatase are independent prognostic variables. These

Table 3. The natural course of PBC – AMA profiles

Group	*n*	*Antibody constellation*	*Bilirubin > 1.5 mg/dl (%)*
A	74	anti-M9+	1
B	211	anti-M9+ and/or anti-M2	6
C	176	anti-M2/-M4+ and/or anti-M8+ (ELISA)	39
D	89	as C, ELISA+ and CFT+	44

From Reference 31

models may be helpful in the timing of liver transplantation. Thus, they are useful only for patients with advanced disease[16].

The imprecision of the prognostic models may be due to the fact that they have used data from just one time-point during an often long course of individual patient's disease. Therefore, serial determinations of bilirubin and also of quantitative liver function tests (galactose-elimination capacity (GEC)) were used. Using GEC, the time of death could be predicted with an accuracy of 7 ± 19 months[17]. Other authors used antibody profiles determined at early stages of PBC in order to differentiate between a stable and a progressive nature of the underlying disease[18] (Table 3). In the immediate pretransplant situation, serum bilirubin concentration, plasma creatinine as well as the pretransplant clinical situation seem to reflect the outcome after transplantation.

PRIMARY SCLEROSING CHOLANGITIS (PSC)

PSC is a chronic destructive, fibroinflammatory condition affecting bile ducts of all sizes. The natural history of disease is incompletely understood. However, most would agree that PSC is usually a progressive syndrome, finally leading to liver-related death in a substantial proportion of patients.

Again, as in the case of PBC, PSC may evolve through several sequential phases.

The preclinical stage

In the preclinical stage, patients are virtually undetectable unless evaluated for unspecific abdominal discomfort. Cholestatic liver enzymes can be normal despite cholangiographic evidence of bile duct alterations. Most patients studied had inflammatory bowel disease simultaneously[19].

The sequential phase

The second sequential phase is that of an asymptomatic patient with elevated cholestatic enzymes in the serum. In early reports, about one third of these patients died after a follow-up of 5–7 years following diagnosis[20,21].

Recent data from a large group of asymptomatic Scandinavian patients (92% of them with ulcerative colitis) disclosed that 22% developed symptoms during follow-up (mean 63 months)[22].

The five-year survival of the asymptomatic group was more than 90%. At 16 years after diagnosis, the survival rate of the asymptomatic group was still 70%, showing a surprisingly benign course of PSC. Only 13% of the asymptomatic patients had died or had OLT[22]. In the Mediterranean area, 30% of 117 PSC patients were asymptomatic at diagnosis. Only 36% of the patients had ulcerative colitis. Survival rate was not related to the presence or absence of symptoms. At ten years, the survival rate was 74%. Thus, PSC in Italy mainly follows a benign course[23]. Also, in a recent study from Norway, no major differences could be observed in the prognosis of symptomatic vs. asymptomatic patients; 99% of patients had inflammatory bowel disease, and a median survival of around 15 years was found[24]. These data are in contrast to results from the US: of 45 asymptomatic patients, fourteen (31%) developed liver failure during follow-up (mean 75.2 months). Of these patients, 82% had ulcerative colitis and 54% developed symptomatic PSC. Compared with matched controls, a significantly diminished survival was noted, regardless of the starting point (suspected evidence of liver disease and diagnosis of liver disease)[25].

The symptomatic phase

In this phase, patients exhibit a variety of hepatobiliary symptoms (fatigue, fever, pruritus, abdominal pain etc.). In some studies, development of symptoms seems to worsen the prognosis substantially. Of 29 patients, 41% died or developed liver failure requiring OLT during a mean follow-up of 6.3 years[26].

In a large cohort of 137 symptomatic patients, 45% died or developed liver failure during a mean follow-up of 6.2 years[20]. The survival rate in 171 symptomatic Scandinavian patients was 25% at 16 years[22].

Taken together, the prognosis of patients with PSC differs remarkably in reported series from different countries. Moreover, endpoints vary and the proportions of symptomatic to asymptomatic patients differ largely in most series. It is generally believed, however, that asymptomatic patients with PBC have a more favourable prognosis: among 137 symptomatic patients, liver-related death occurred after a follow-up of 6.0 years (mean; range 2.7–15.5 years) in 37%, as compared to 8% among 37 asymptomatic patients[20]. The ten-year actuarial survival was calculated to be 93% in asymptomatic and 47% in symptomatic patients[27]. Obviously, there is no relationship between the course of PSC and that of accompanying inflammatory bowel disease[28]. However, survival curves based on histological stage at entry showed that survival decreased with increasing stage on liver biopsy[20].

The post-transplant phase

For patients who develop end-stage PSC, OLT is the only effective treatment modality currently available. In a recent study, 5-year survival was 87.9%[28]. However, no cholangiocarcinoma was identified at the time of OLT in this group of patients. Therefore, survival rates following OLT must be regarded as very good in this group of patients. It should be stressed that colon cancer represents the most frequent cause of death in PSC patients following OLT. This complication may develop rapidly in patients receiving immunosuppression. Close endoscopic supervision, therefore, is mandatory.

Is there recurrence of PSC in the transplanted liver?

pANCA persist (with reduced titres) in PSC patients after OLT. These autoantibodies, however, are not associated with histological evidence of disease recurrence[29]. Histologically, biliary obstructive features and fibrous cholangitis were more common in allografts of PSC patients than in controls. Therefore, it has been concluded that PSC may recur in the liver allograft[30]. However, although PSC does occur in the graft, it is still unclear whether this is disease recurrence or merely a secondary sclerosing cholangitis upon biliary problems and/or hypoxaemia.

Factors predictive of prognosis in PSC

As in the case of PBC, prognostic indices using the Cox multivariate model have been published. The Mayo Clinic found that high age, high bilirubin, low haemoglobin and advanced histological stage are significantly associated with survival[20].

Again, as in the case of PBC, serum bilirubin levels alone could probably be used as a 'poor man's prognostic parameter' also for PSC patients (Table 1). Still unresolved is the question of early detection of cholangiocarcinoma, a major threat to patients with long-standing PSC. Regular non-invasive evaluation of the biliary tree with magnetic resonance cholangiography could be an option for the near future.

References

1. Mitchison HC, Bassendine MF, Hendrick A et al. Positive antimitochondrial antibody but normal alkaline phosphatase: Is this primary biliary cirrhosis? Hepatology. 1986;6:1278–84.
2. Metcalf JV, Mitchison HC, Palmer JM, Jones DE, Bassendine MF, James OFW. Natural history of early primary biliary cirrhosis. Lancet. 1996;348:1399–402.
3. Roll J, Boyer JL, Barry D, Klatskin G. The prognostic importance of clinical and histologic features on asymptomatic and symptomatic primary biliary cirrhosis. N Engl J Med. 1983;308:1–7.
4. Kapelman B, Schaffner F. The natural history of primary biliary cirrhosis. Semin Liver Dis. 1981;1:273–81.
5. Mahl TC, Shockcor W, Boyer JL. Primary biliary cirrhosis: survival of a large cohort of symptomatic and asymptomatic patients followed for 24 years. J Hepatol. 1994;20:707–13.
6. Beswick DR, Klatskin G, Boyer JL. Asymptomatic primary biliary cirrhosis: a progress report on long-term follow-up and natural history. Gastroenterology. 1985;89:267–1.
7. James O, Watson AJ, Macklon AF. Primary biliary cirrhosis – a revised clinical spectrum. Lancet. 1981;1:1278–81.
8. Balasubramaniam K, Grambsch PM, Wiesner RH, Lindor KD, Dickson ER. Diminished survival in asymptomatic primary biliary cirrhosis. Gastroenterology. 1990;98:1567–71.
9. Mitchison HC, Luvey MR, Kelly PJ. Symptom development and prognosis in primary biliary cirrhosis: a study in two centers. Gastroenterology. 1990;99:778–82.
10. Nyberg A, Lööf L. Primary biliary cirrhosis: clinical features and outcome, with special reference to asymptomatic disease. Scand J Gastroenterol. 1989;24:57–61.
11. Tzakis AG, Carcassonne C, Todo S. Liver transplantation. Semin Liv Dis. 1989;9:144–8.

12. Esquivel CO, Van Thiel DH, Demetris AJ. Transplantation for primary biliary cirrhosis. Gastroenterology. 1989;94:1207–5.
13. Balan V, Batts KP, Porayoko MK. Histological evidence for recurrence of primary biliary cirrhosis after liver transplantation. Hepatology. 1993;18:1392–6.
14. Hubscher SG, Elias E, Buckels JAC. Primary biliary cirrhosis. Histologic evidence of disease recurrence after liver transplantation. J Hepatol. 1993;18:173–80.
15. Shapiro JM, Smith H, Schaffner F. Serum bilirubin: a prognostic factor in primary biliary cirrhosis. Gut. 1979;20:137–40.
16. Kaplan MM. Primary biliary cirrhosis. N Engl J Med. 1996;335:1570–81.
17. Reichen J, Widmer T, Cotting J. Accurate prediction of death by serial determination of galactose elimination capacity in primary biliary cirrhosis: a comparison with the Mayo model. Hepatology. 1991;14:504–10.
18. Klein R, Klöppel G, Garbe V, Fintelmann V, Berg PA. Antimitochondrial antibody profiles determined at early stages of primary biliary cirrhosis differentiate between a benign and a progressive course of the disease. J Hepatol. 1991;12:21–7.
19. Balasubramaniam K, Wiesner RH, LaRusso NF. Can serum alkaline phosphatase levels be normal in primary sclerosing cholangitis? Gastroenterology. 1987;92(Abstract):1303.
20. Wiesner RH, Grambsch PM, Dickson ER et al. Primary sclerosing cholangitis: natural history, prognostic factors and survival analysis. Hepatology. 1989;10:430–6.
21. Chapman RW, Arborgh BA, Rhodes JM et al. Primary sclerosing cholangitis: a review of its clinical features, cholangiography, and hepatic histology. Gut. 1980;21:870–7.
22. Broomé U, Olsson R, Lööf L et al. Natural history and prognostic factors in 305 Swedish patients with primary sclerosing cholangitis. Gut. 1996;38:610–15.
23. Okolicsanyi L, Fabris L, Viaggi N, Carulli N, Podda M, Ricci G and the Italian PSC Study Group. Primary sclerosing cholangitis: clinical presentation, natural history and prognostic variables: an Italian multicentre study. Eur J Gastroenterol Hepatol. 1996;8:685–91.
24. Schrumpf E, Abdelnoor M, Fausa O, Elgjo K, Jenssen E, Kolmannskog F. Risk factors in primary sclerosing cholangitis. J Hepatol. 1994;21:1061–6.
25. Porayko MK, Wiesner RH, Larusso NF et al. Patients with asymptomatic primary sclerosing cholangitis frequently have progressive disease. Gastroenterology. 1990;98:1594–602.
26. Lebovics E, Palmer M, Woo J. Outcome of primary sclerosing cholangitis: analysis of long-term observation of 38 patients. Arch Intern Med. 1987;147:729–31.
27. Vierling JM. Hepatobiliary complications of ulcerative colitis and Crohn's disease. In Zakim D, Boyer Th.D (Eds.) Hepatology. W.B. Saunders; 1996:1366.
28. Lee YM, Kaplan M. Primary sclerosing cholangitis. N Engl J Med. 1995;6:924–33.
29. Haagsma EB, Mulder AH, Gouw AS. Neutrophil cytoplasmic autoantibodies after liver transplantation in patients with primary sclerosing cholangitis. J Hepatol. 1993;19:8–12.
30. Harrison RF, Davies MH, Neuberger JM, Hubscher SG. Fibrous and obliterative cholangitis in liver allografts: evidence of recurrent primary sclerosing cholangitis? Hepatology. 1994;20: 356–61.
31. Berg PA, Klein R. Mitochondrial antigen/antibody systems in primary biliary cirrhosis: revisited. Liver. 1995;15:281–92.

9
Morphological aspects of overlap syndromes

H.P. DIENES, G. GERKEN, A. LOHSE, P. SCHIRMACHER and K.H. MEYER ZUM BÜSCHENFELDE

INTRODUCTION

The overlap syndromes in autoimmune liver diseases designate the simultaneous occurrence of autoimmune hepatitis (AIH) and primary biliary cirrhosis (PBC) and autoimmune hepatitis and primary sclerosing cholangitis (PSC) whereas the association of PBC with PSC has, so far, not been reported. In the diagnosis of a genuine overlap syndrome (OLS), all criteria of either disease have to be fulfilled; otherwise the disease has to be termed according to the major disorder with the component only of the other disease.

AIH/PBC OLS

According to a unified concept of autoimmune hepatitis[1], the same immunological mechanism may attack hepatocytes and/or bile duct epithelia and induce hepatitis or PBC respectively, thus implying that a simultaneous manifestation of AIH and PBC may not be an uncommon event. However, a review of the experience and the analysis of the daily pathological practice shows the contrary: OLS of AIH and PBC are still the subject of case reports[2].

In order to delineate the OLS of AIH and PBC, the two disease components have to be defined precisely. The entity of AIH presents as a multifaceted disease, encompassing different subtypes according to autoantibodies[3]. Although modern techniques in serology have improved the sensitivity and specificity of test systems, in the individual patient the diagnosis may be difficult to confirm and seronegative cases of AIH seem to exist[4].

Histopathology may display characteristic but by no means pathognomonic lesions[5]. In the active phase of the disease, piecemeal necroses are conspicuous and may expand to confluent periportal necrosis with parenchymal collapse. Preserved hepatocytes in that area may undergo microascinar transformation. Lobular necrosis and inflammatory activity are more prominent than in viral hepatitis. Bile

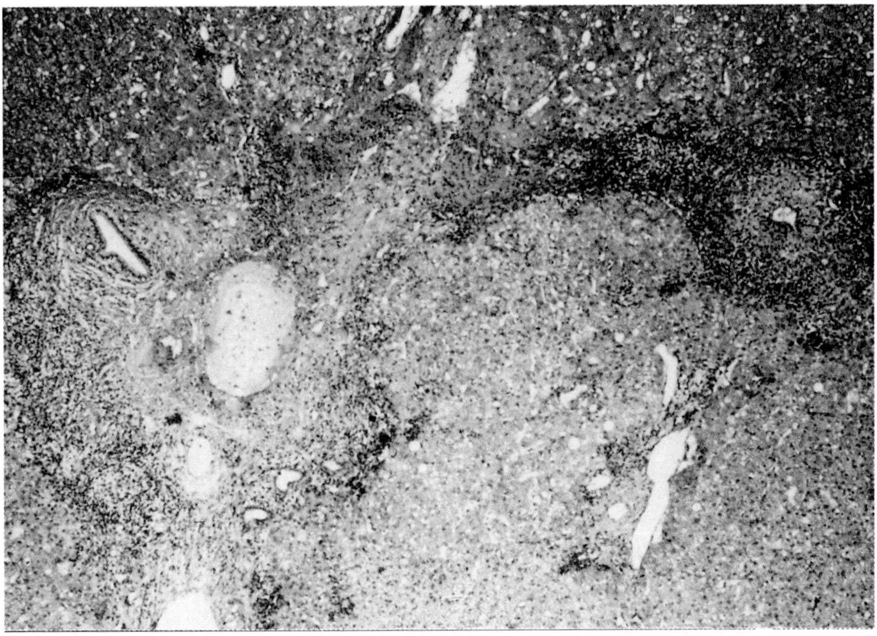

Figure 1. Liver from a patient with AIH-PBC overlap syndrome: portal tracts are enlarged and connected by active septa. Besides bile duct destruction there is a significant inflammation in the lobules (H&E, ×60)

ducts may be involved to a variable extent; however, in contrast to PBC, there is no overt destruction of the basement membranes, epithelioid granulomas are absent and only the small bile ducts may be affected.

The diagnosis of AIH has to be established on the basis of clinical course, serology, histopathology and response to steroids according to a recommended scoring system[3]. PBC seems to present, in contrast to AIH, as a disease well defined by clinical symptoms, autoantibodies to mitochondrial antigens type II and high titres of IgM in the serum. Histopathology reveals lesions of medium-sized bile ducts that are regarded as pathognomonic of the disease: the basement membranes are disrupted and lymphocytes may invade the epithelia that undergo necrosis. Epithelioid granulomas are often abutted onto the bile ducts. Piecemeal necroses may occur but are not essential to the disease. The involvement of the lobules in PBC consists of mild inflammatory infiltrates but does not include obvious hepatocellular necrosis.

The AIH/PBC overlap syndrome was first described by Popper and Schaffner[6]. The coincidence of PBC and fully developed AIH has been documented at the clinical, serological and histological level only in few cases[2,7–10]. A report[11] on a larger cohort of patients with ‘mixed types of chronic aggressive hepatitis and PBC’ was published in the late seventies. The common denominator of this group were autoantibodies to a ‘CAH/PBC mixed-type’ antigen. Of the 13 patients, 7 would have met strict criteria of OLS by clinical symptoms, serology and histopathology. It is remarkable that none of the patients of the mixed CAH/PBC type

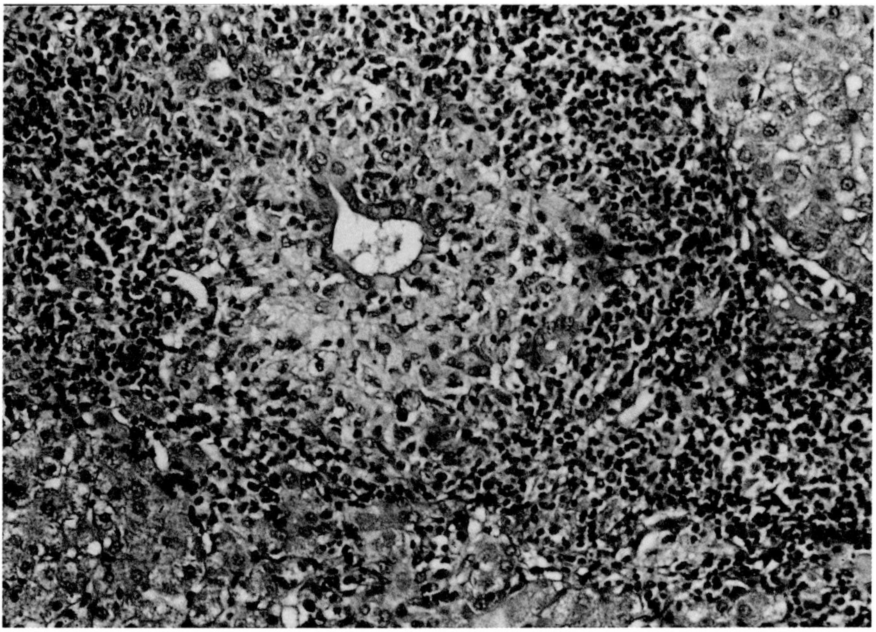

Figure 2. Same biopsy as in Figure 1: in the centre, there is a bile duct undergoing destruction within a granuloma. Note abundant piecemeal necroses (H&E, ×240)

had AMA type 2 autoantibodies. In the 7 cases that showed criteria of OLS also by histopathology, bile duct lesions with granuloma formation and necroinflammatory changes in the lobules were present. The assessment of a genuine AIH/PBC OLS has to meet the following criteria at clinicoserological and histopathological levels.

(1) Clinical and biochemical evidence for dynamic hepatitis with autoantibodies according to an interactioned group. Additionally AMAs type 2 and signs of cholestasis as elevation of AP and bilirubin.

(2) Histopathology must show criteria of substantial necroinflammatory lesions in liver parenchyma, piecemeal necrosis for the AIH component and portal inflammation, bile duct damage with loss of epithelia and disruption of basement membranes for PBC (Fig. 1). Epithelioid granulomas belong to the morphological diagnosis (Fig. 2) but may be missed in a small biopsy.

So far, the dynamic evolution of the course of each of the two diseases has not been carefully evaluated or delineated. Most studies report simultaneous occurrence of both diseases; only Duclos-Vallée et al.[2] describe a patient who suffered from AIH before PBC developed. Both diseases were successfully treated with CyA. The immunopathological basis of the AIH/PBC overlap syndrome has yet to be analysed. In AIH, the hepatocytes seem to be the targets for the cell-mediated immune attack whereas, in PBC, bile duct epithelia are assumed to play this role; however, it has not been investigated whether, in the OLS, instead of one there

Table 1. Case reports of patients with AIH/PSC OLS

References	*Age and sex of patients*	*Autoantibodies*	*Course**
Minuk et al. (1988)[13]	30, m	SMA	PCH-AIH
	18, f	ANA, SMA	AIH-PSC
Rabinovitz et al. (1992)[17]	30, m	ANA, SMA	AIH-PSC
Lawrence et al. (1994)[14]	39, m	SMA	AIH-PSC
Gohlke et al. (1996)[12]	19, m	ANA SMA pANCA	AIH-PSC
	28, m	ANA pANCA	AIH-PSC
	18, m	ANA SMA pANCA	AIH-PSC

*PSC-AIH = PSC preceded AIH; AIH-PSC = AIH and PSC were diagnosed simultaneously

are two types of target cells or whether the pathways leading to the overlapping are different.

AIH/PSC OLS

The other category of autoimmune OLS of liver diseases covers the combination of AIH and PSC. The incidence of this type of OLS is less common than that of AIH/PBC. Only few case reports have been published[12]; these are summarized in Table 1. The mean age of patients is lower than that for AIH/PBC OLS. Most of them are males and only Minuk et al.[13] have reported on two female patients. The spectrum of autoantibodies includes SMA, ANA and pANCA. In most cases, AIH precedes the manifestation of PSC which may emerge when the patients are under steroid therapy. Histopathology of AIH/PSC OLS includes the necroinflammatory parenchymal damage of AIH with dense portal inflammatory infiltration and piecemeal necrosis on the one hand and the simultaneous manifestation of sclerosing cholangitis with periductular fibrosis, thickening of basement membranes and degenerative changes of the epithelia on the other hand. Although morphology of bile ducts in the PSC phase may be diagnostic with the periductular fibrotic cuff, degenerative changes of bile duct epithelia and hyalin thickening of basement membranes, the diagnosis in this OLS should be confirmed by ERCP. Lawrence et al.[14] have termed this condition 'inflammatory PSC'; however, the course and response to steroid treatment of the hepatitis on the one hand and the development of the cholangitis on the other reflect the manifestation of two different diseases.

Recently, another variant of OLS of AIH and PSC has been described[15]. The postinfantile giant cell hepatitis is a progressive form of chronic hepatitis with an obscure aetiology[15]. There is, however, substantial evidence that, in combi-nation with PSC, it is of autoimmune origin. The report by Protzer et al.[15] showed that the main criteria of AIH were present in these patients who simultaneously suffered from PSC. All patients had autoantibodies as SMA, ANA, and/or anti-asialoglycoprotein receptor. They were of typical HLA-A1, B8 DR3/4 haplotype

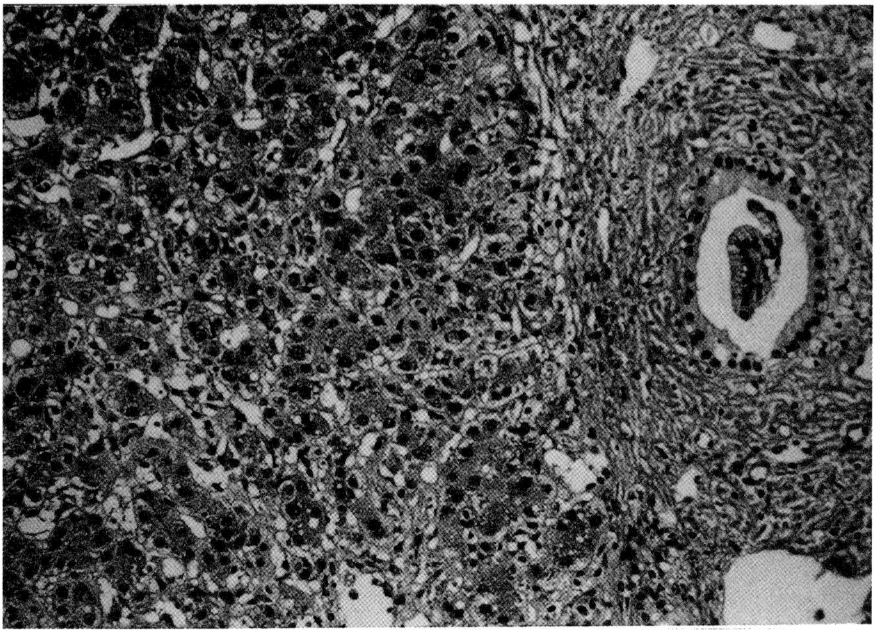

Figure 3. Liver biopsy from a patient with AIH-PSC overlap syndrome: A medium-sized bile duct shows typical fibrotic cuff with degenerative changes of bile duct epithelia. In the lobule, marked sinusoidal infiltration is obvious (H&E, ×360)

and, in all patients, the hepatitis responded to steroid treatment. Histopathology displayed a conspicuous giant cell formation of the hepatocytes in up to 30% of the parenchymal cells. There was severe cholestasis with bile pigment in hepatocytes and casts in the dilated bile canaliculi. Bile ducts showed typical periductal fibrosis and degenerative changes of epithelia. The diagnosis was confirmed by endoscopic retrograde cholangiography. Combined treatment with steroids and UDCA was successful.

It is difficult to explain the simultaneous development of AIH and PSC by a unified concept of immunology, since the mechanisms of bile duct loss in PSC are, so far, poorly understood. At least, the underlying problem does not seem to be a cell-mediated immune reaction with bile duct epithelia as targets[16]. There is evidence, however, that excess production of the cytokine TGFβ1 may play a role in both diseases.

SUMMARY

The main overlap syndromes of autoimmune liver diseases are AIH/PBC and AIH/PSC, whose diagnosis must be confirmed at the clinicoserological and histopathological level. In the OLS, histopathology reflects features of both diseases that may be expressed to different degrees and run separate courses of their own. In AIH/PBC, morphology is in accordance with the concept that both hepatocytes and bile duct epithelia may become target cells of a lymphocyte-mediated immune attack, whereas, in AIH/PSC, the underlying mechanisms are still obscure. For AIH/PSC overlap syndrome, a special variant has been described with the AIH presenting as postinfantile giant cell hepatitis.

References

1. Doniach D, Walker JD. A unified concept of autoimmune hepatitis. Lancet. 1969;1:813–15.
2. Duclos-Vallée JC, Hadengue A, Ganne-Carrié N, Robin E, Degott C, Erlinger S. Primary biliary cirrhosis – autoimmune hepatitis overlap syndrome. Dig Dis Sci. 1995;40:1069–73.
3. Johnsohn PJ, McFarlane IG. Meeting report: International Autoimmune Hepatitis Group. Hepatology. 1993;18:998–1005.
4. Meyer zum Büschenfelde KH, Dienes HP. Autoimmune hepatitis. Definition – classification – histopathology – immunopathogenesis. Virch Arch. 1996;429:1–12.
5. Dienes HP, Popper H, Manns M et al. Histologic features in autoimmune hepatitis. Z Gastroenterol. 1989;27:325–30.
6. Popper H, Schaffner F. Nonsuppurative destructive chronic cholangitis and chronic hepatitis. In: Popper H, Schaffner P, eds. Progress in Liver Diseases, Vol III. New York: Grune & Stratton; 1970: 336–54.
7. Carrougher JG, Schaffer RT, Canales LI, Goofman ZD. A 33-year old woman with an autoimmune syndrome. Semin Liv Dis. 1991;11:256–62.
8. Geubel AP, Baggestoss SH, Summerskill WHJ. Responses to treatment can differentiate chronic active liver disease with cholangitic features from primary biliary cirrhosis. Gastroenterology. 1976;71:444–9.
9. Okuna T, Yoshifumi S, Okanoue T, Takino T. Chronic active hepatitis with histological features of primary biliary cirrhosis. Dig Dis Sci. 1987;32:775–9.
10. Saeki R, Kaneko S, Terasaki S et al. Mixed types of chronic active hepatitis and primary biliary cirrhosis associated with the anti-phospholipid antibody syndrome: A case report. Hepato-Gastroenterology. 1993;40:499–501.
11. Klöppel G, Seifert G, Lindner H, Dammermann R, Sack HJ, Berg PA. Histopathological features in mixed types of chronic aggressive hepatitis and primary biliary cirrhosis. Correlations of liver histology with mitochondrial antibodies of different specificity. Virch Arch. 1977;373:143–60.
12. Gohlke F, Lohse AW, Dienes HP et al. Evidence of an overlap syndrome of autoimmune hepatitis and primary sclerosing cholangitis. J Hepatol. 1996;24:699–705.
13. Minuk GY, Sutherland LR, Pappas SC et al. Autoimmune chronic active hepatitis (lupoid hepatitis) and primary sclerosing cholangitis in two young adult females. Can J Gastroenterol. 1988;2:22–7.
14. Lawrence SP, Sherman KE, Lawson JM, Goodman ZD. A 39 year old man with chronic hepatitis. Semin Liv Dis. 1994;14:97–105.
15. Protzer U, Dienes HP, Bianchi L et al. Post infantile giant cell hepatitis in patients with primary sclerosing cholangitis and autoimmune hepatitis. Liver. 1996;16:274–82.
16. Dienes HP, Lohse AW, Gerken G et al. Bile duct epithelia as target cells in primary biliary cirrhosis (PBC) and primary sclerosing cholangitis (PSC). Virch Arch. 1997 [accepted for publication].
17. Rabinovitz M, Demetris AJ, Bou-Abboud DF, Van Thiel DH. Simultaneous occurrence of primary sclerosing cholangitis and autoimmune chronic active hepatitis in a patient with ulcerative colitis. Dig Dis Sci. 1992;37:1606–11.

10
Distinction between autoimmune and viral liver diseases

G. GERKEN

INTRODUCTION

In most instances, autoimmune hepatitis can easily be distinguished from chronic viral hepatitis. However, the occurrence of autoantibodies in viral hepatitis has raised the question of differential diagnosis of the two diseases (Table 1). Indeed, the clear distinction between viral and autoimmune hepatitis is of important clinical relevance regarding treatment of the patients (Table 2). Whereas interferon-α may lead to severe deterioration of patients with autoimmune hepatitis, the therapeutic use of corticosteroids is ineffective or may be deleterious in patients with virus-induced liver diseases.

Viruses are involved in autoimmune diseases on the basis of different findings. First, autoimmune responses are made *de novo* or those already present are enhanced by concomitant infection by different viruses. Secondly, both acute and persistent viral infections can induce, accelerate or enhance autoimmune responses and cause autoimmune disease. Viruses also can influence the release of lympho-

Table 1. Liver autoreactions in viral hepatitis

Virus	*Autoantibodies*
HAV	SMA, LSP, ASGPR
HBV	LSP, ASGPR, ANA, SMA
HCV	LKM, ASGPR, AMA, ANA, SMA, GOR
HDV	LKM, LSP, ASGPR

Table 2. Differential therapy

Viral hepatitis	Interferon
Autoimmune hepatitis	Immunosuppression
Viral hepatitis with autoantibodies	Interferon
Coincidence of viral and autoimmune hepatitis	Immunosuppression

Table 3. Definition of autoimmune hepatitis

Hypergammaglobulinaemia	+3
Autoantibodies	
ANA, SMA, LKM-1	+3
SLA, ASGPR, LC, LP, HHPM	+2
AMA	−2
Female sex (80–90%)	+2
Benefit from immunosuppression	+2
Genetics – B8-DR3 or DR4	+1
HBsAg, IgM and HAV	−3

kines and monokines. Third, molecular mimicry between pathogens and human cell proteins may play a role in the induction of autoimmune mechanisms.

In this brief overview, we will discuss autoimmune phenomena in viral hepatitis.

COEXISTENCE OF VIRAL AND AUTOIMMUNE LIVER DISEASE

The classical syndrome of autoimmune hepatitis is clearly characterized by a certain age, sex and HLA association as well as by the occurrence of different autoantibodies[1,2] (Table 3). Histological features can also be useful in distinguishing autoimmune hepatitis, chronic viral hepatitis type B and type C[3]. Immunogenetic markers, including HLA B8, DR3 and DR4, are significantly more common in autoimmune hepatitis. In a recent study from Lohse et al.[4], we have compared 352 patients with autoimmune liver disease and 507 patients with viral hepatitis for diagnostic characteristics as well as for evidence of an aetiological connection. Nineteen per cent of patients with chronic hepatitis C and 14% of patients with chronic hepatitis B had significant titres of autoantibodies (ANA, SMA, LKM). SLA autoantibodies were found exclusively in patients with autoimmune liver disease. LKM autoantibodies were found in only one of these 201 HCV patients. Evidence of past or present hepatitis B virus and past hepatitis A virus infection was most common in the hepatitis C virus patients and least common in autoimmune hepatitis. Twenty-eight of the 352 patients with autoimmune liver disease tested positive in the second-generation anti-HCV assay but only 5 patients were additionally positive in confirmatory anti-HCV test and, only in these, could HCV-RNA be detected. Autoimmune hepatitis patients had significantly higher serum transaminase levels, higher serum IgG levels and were significantly more positive for the expression of HLA B8, HLA DR3 and HLA DR4.

Taken together, distinction between autoimmune hepatitis and viral hepatitis C can be made reliably on clinical and laboratory grounds. Our data clearly show that the link between hepatitis type A, B or C and autoimmune liver diseases is rarely confirmed. False positive anti-HCV ELISA results are found in about 5% of patients with autoimmune liver disease. True HCV infection is a rare event. Autoantibodies could be found frequently in both hepatitis B and hepatitis C and were therefore only of limited help in the differential diagnosis. Actually, we have also tested the connection between the newly described HGV/GBV-C virus and patients with autoimmune hepatitis. In accordance with Heringlake et al.[5], HGV/GBV-C does not play any major role in autoimmune hepatitis (Table 4). Finally,

Table 4. HGV-RNA in hepatitis C and autoimmune hepatitis ($n = 163$)

	HGV positive
Hepatitis C	
Genotype 3a	15/56 (27%)
Genotype 1a	2/26 (8%)
Genotype 1b	2/32 (6%)
Autoimmune hepatitis	3/49 (6%)
Subtype I	1/18
Subtype II	2/15
Subtype III	0/15

Table 5. Autoantibodies in HCV-infection

Autoantibody	*Percentage*	*Reference*
Anti-nuclear (ANA)	6.9	4
Anti-smooth muscle (SMA)	14.8	4
Anti-soluble liver antigen (SLA)	10	18
Anti-asialoglycoprotein receptor (ASGPR)	13	15
Anti-liver/kidney microsomes (LKM)	5	19
Anti-GOR	80	20

patients with chronic viral hepatitis typically have much lower autoantibody titres than those with autoimmune hepatitis. Furthermore, the immunodominant epitopes of the autoantigens may be different between viral and autoimmune hepatitis. This has been recently suggested, not only for microsomal antigens, but also for epitopes of the asialoglycoprotein receptor[6,7].

VIRUS-INDUCED AUTOIMMUNITY IN HEPATITIS

Importantly, HCV infection has been closely associated with seropositivity for anti-LKM autoantibodies and this association has generated speculation that HCV may be the aetiological agent of type 2 autoimmune hepatitis (Table 5). LKM autoantibodies were initially described as a diagnostic marker for a second subgroup of autoimmune hepatitis. The major autoantigen recognized by LKM autoantibodies in autoimmune hepatitis was identified as cytochrome P_{450} dbl[8]. These LKM autoantibodies were labelled LKM-1 to distinguish them from LKM-2 autoantibodies reactive with a different cytochrome isoenzyme and associated with tielenic-acid-induced hepatitis and LKM-3 autoantibodies associated with Delta hepatitis[9]. LKM-positive hepatitis appears to be particularly common in Italy where hepatitis C infection has higher prevalence[10]. This is in accordance with our patients where we showed HCV infection in 9 out of 22 LKM-positive sera[4]. Clinically the two groups, LKM-positive autoimmune hepatitis and LKM-positive hepatitis C virus infection, respectively, were very distinct with no evidence of genuine autoimmune disease in the HCV-positive LKM-positive patients, most of whom showed a good response to interferon treatment. Lunel *et al.*[6] presented data on a series of 83 LKM-1-positive patients from France. Seventy-seven per cent were anti-HCV positive by ELISA and 49% were con-

Table 6. Characteristics of patients with LKM-1 positive chronic hepatitis with or without HCV

	HCV-negative	*HCV-positive*
Age	Young	Older
Sex	Female	No predominance
SGPT	↑↑↑	↑
LKM-1 titre	+++	+
Immunosuppression	+++	?
IFN	No indication	(+)
DR3	++	+
C4A-Q0	+	+

firmed to be truly positive by RIBA. HCV-RNA could be isolated in all the RIBA-positive patients. Taken together, patients with autoimmune-type LKM-positive hepatitis are found to be younger, female and have more active disease in older patients[11] (Table 6). Furthermore, there is evidence that the epitopes recognized by hepatitis-C-associated LKM-1 autoantibodies are different from those recognized by sera from LKM-positive autoimmune hepatitis. Although in both conditions the LKM autoantibodies detected mostly show binding to the cytochrome P_{450} isoenzyme 2D6, the exact peptide specificity of these antibodies in patients is different with autoimmune hepatitis compared with hepatitis C[12]. In addition, some autoantibodies in chronic hepatitis C giving the LKM in fluorescence pattern do not react with recombinant cytochrome 2D6, suggesting that they recognize another isoenzyme. Furthermore, anti-GOR antibodies against an antigen isolated from an HCV-positive chimpanzee liver and identified as a host-encoded antigen with no recognizable relationship to HCV-encoded proteins can be found in most patients with HCV-related hepatitis but are only rarely found in autoimmune diseases or other liver diseases. The pathogenesis and significance of these antibodies is still elusive. We have found anti-GOR reactivity to be useful in the differential diagnosis of patients with LKM-positive liver disease[13]. Patients with autoimmune positive LKM hepatitis did not show any anti-GOR reactivity.

INTERFERON-INDUCED AUTOIMMUNITY IN VIRAL HEPATITIS

Interferon-α has been shown to be a promising therapeutic approach to the treatment of chronic viral hepatitis. However, several reports have described the development of autoantibodies during and after interferon therapy. Therefore, the possibility exists that interferon therapy in chronic viral hepatitis may induce autoimmune responses that may potentiate the liver disease. In an earlier study from our group by Mayet *et al.*[14], we were able to show that most patients develop autoantibodies during or after interferon-α treatment. In general, autoantibodies to ANA appeared first, followed by antibodies to SMA. Finally, antibodies to endocrine cells arose. Which factors did determine the appearance of autoantibodies and their sequence of detection remains unclear. In conclusion, this study did not show any evidence that interferon-α therapy of chronic type B hepatitis induced autoimmune liver disease. Antibodies associated with other autoimmune disorders appeared and therefore interferon-α therapy may be harmful to patients with a pre-existing non-hepatic autoimmune disorder. In view of this, we think that interferon-α treatment should be used with caution in patients with autoimmune conditions, especially those who may have autoimmune liver diseases. In a further study by Treichel *et al.*[15], the occurrence and titre of anti-human ASGPR autoantibodies were characterized in sera from patients with autoimmune as well as viral hepatitis and additionally, after initiation of either immunosuppressive or recombinant interferon-α treatment, respectively. In this study we showed that, in viral hepatitis, anti-human ASGPR autoantibodies were found much less frequently, in lower titres and without association with the disease activity as assessed by histological and by biochemical parameters. In patients with chronic hepatitis B as well as with chronic hepatitis C, an induction of anti-human ASGPR with a maximum titre of 1:600 was found which was only transient in 4 of 5 patients during interferon-α treatment. Interestingly, immunoglobulin classification revealed IgG and IgM classes in both cases with untreated autoimmune hepatitis and viral-induced hepatitis exhibiting mainly IgG-2 subclass in autoimmune, and IgG-4 in viral, hepatitis. High titres of anti-human ASGPR in autoimmune hepatitis were exclusively of the IgG type in contrast to anti-human ASGPR in chronic viral hepatitis which exhibited both IgG and IgM class anti-human ASGPR despite lower titre values. Thus, these results clearly indicate different patterns of anti-human ASGPR occurrence, titre and immunoglobulin class in patients suffering from either autoimmune hepatitis or viral-induced hepatitis. This suggests different pathways of induction and perpetuation of autoantibody formation in inflammatory liver disease in man.

SUMMARY

Differentiation between autoimmune hepatitis with concomitant viral liver disease on the one hand and viral liver disease with induction of autoantibodies on the other has to be carefully made since therapeutic strategies differ widely (Table 7)[16,17]. In the few cases of diagnostic uncertainty as well as in those patients with coincidental hepatitis C and autoimmune hepatitis, the therapeutic choice should primarily be a trial of immunosuppressive therapy. Firstly, the inadvertent administration of interferon in autoimmune hepatitis can be very detrimental. Secondly, the prognosis of untreated autoimmune hepatitis is generally very poor while the prognosis of hepatitis given adequate immunosuppressive therapy is excellent. Bearing this in mind, the suspicion of autoimmune hepatitis should dictate the initial therapeutic choice. In those very rare cases of diagnostic uncertainty and non-responsiveness to immunosuppressive therapy in a patient with a mixed clinical picture and definite proof of viral infection, interferon can then be used in a subsequent therapeutic trial but requires frequent close monitoring.

Finally, hepatitis C virus as well as hepatitis G virus has been rather convincingly excluded as a major cause of autoimmune hepatitis. Therefore, the search for a trigger will have to continue and it is open to speculation whether it is an infectious agent, an environmental agent or an intrinsic event in the patient's immune system. Autoantibodies in viral liver diseases appear to be an expression of a generalized immunoactivation by cytokines.

Table 7. Antibodies and treatment responses in chronic non-B hepatitis

	ANA	*LKM*	*SLA*	*SMA*	*AMA*	*ASGPR*	*Anti-GOR*	*Anti-HCV*	*Steroid response*	*Interferon response*
Classical AIH	+/(+)	–	–	(+)/+	–	+/(+)	–	–	+	–
LKM-positive AIH	–	+	–	–	–	+/(+)	–	–	+	–
SLA-positive AIH	–	–	+	+/–	+/–	+/(+)	–	–	+	–
Overlap PBC/AIH	+	–	(+)	(+)	+	+	–	–	(+)/+	–
Primary biliary cirrhosis (PBC)	(+)	–	–	–	+	(+)	–	–	(+)	–
Cryptogenic hepatitis – AIH type	–	–	–	–	–	(+)	–	–	+	–
Cryptogenic hepatitis – viral type	–	–	–	–	–	–	–	–	–	+
LKM-positive chronic hepatitis C	–	+	–	–	–	–	+	+	–	(+)
Chronic hepatitis C	(+)	–	–	(+)	–	–	+	+	–	+
Chronic hepatitis G	–	–	–	–	–	–	–	+/–	–	+

References

1. Meyer zum Büschenfelde K-H, Dienes H-P. Autoimmune hepatitis. Definition – classification – histopathology – immunopathogenesis. Virchows Arch. 1996;429:1–12.
2. Johnson PJ, McFarlain IG. Meeting report: International Autoimmune Hepatitis Group. Hepatology. 1993;18:998–1005.
3. Desmet V, Gerber MA, Hoofnagel JH, Manns MP, Scheuer P. Classification of chronic hepatitis: diagnosis, grading and staging. Hepatology. 1994;19:1513–20.
4. Lohse AW, Gerken G, Mohr H et al. Relation between autoimmune liver diseases and viral hepatitis: clinical and serological characteristics in 859 patients. Z Gastroenterol. 1995;33:527–33.
5. Heringlake S, Tillmann HL, Cordes-Temme P, Trautwein C, Hunsmann G, Manns MP. GBV-C/HGV is not the major cause of autoimmune hepatitis. J Hepatol. 1996;25:980–4.
6. Lunel FN, Abuaf L, Frangeul L et al. Liver/kidney microsome antibody type 1 and hepatitis C virus infection. Hepatology. 1992;16:630–6.
7. Treichel U, Gerken G, Meyer zum Büschenfelde K-H. Autoantibodies in chronic hepatitis. In: Thomas L, ed. Labor und Diagnose, 5. Auflage: Med Verlagsgesellschaft Marburg; 1997 [In press].
8. Manns MP, Johnson EF, Griffin KJ, Tan EM, Sullivan KF. The major antigen of liver kidney microsomal autoantibodies in idiopathic immune hepatitis is cytochrome p450 dbl. J Clin Invest. 1989;83:1066–72.
9. Phillip T, Straub P, Durazzo M, Tukey RH, Manns MP. Molecular analysis of autoantigens in hepatitis D. J Hepatol. 1995;22(Suppl.):132–135.
10. Lenzi M, Johnson PJ, McFarlane IG et al. Antibodies to hepatitis C virus in autoimmune liver disease: evidence for geographical heterogeneity. Lancet. 1991;338:277–80.
11. Michel G, Ritter A, Gerken G, Meyer zum Büschenfelde K-H, Decker R, Manns M. Anti-GOR and hepatitis C virus in autoimmune liver disease. Lancet. 1992;339:267–9.
12. Klein R, Zanger U, Berg T, Horf U, Berg PA. Anti-LKM Antikörper bei Patienten mit autoimmuner Hepatitis Typ II und Hepatitis C reagieren mit demselben Antigen (Cytochrom p450 2D6), aber erkennen unterschiedliche Epitope. Z Gastroenterol. 1997;35:81A.
13. Löhr H, Gerken G, Michel G, Braun H-B, Meyer zum Büschenfelde K-H. In vitro secretion of anti-GOR protein and anti hepatitis C virus in patients with chronic hepatitis C. Gastroenterology. 1994;107:1443–8.
14. Mayet WJ, Hess G, Gerken G et al. Treatment of chronic hepatitis with recombinant alpha-interferon induces autoantibodies not specific for autoimmune chronic hepatitis. Hepatology. 1989;10:24–8.
15. Treichel U, Gerken G, Rossol S, Poralla Th, Meyer zum Büschenfelde K-H. Autoantibodies against the human asialglycoprotein receptor: effects of therapy in autoimmune and virus-induced chronic hepatitis. J Hepatol. 1993;19:55–63.
16. Treichel U, Meyer zum Büschenfelde K-H, Gerken G. HCV infection and autoimmunity: clinical features, diagnostic tools and therapeutical aspects. Méd Mal Infect. 1995;25:1089–96.
17. Meyer zum Büschenfelde K-H, Lohse AW. Autoimmune hepatitis. N Engl J Med. 1995;333: 1004–5.
18. Czaja AJ, Carpenter HA, Manns MP. Antibodies to SLA, P450 2D6 and mitochondrial complexes in chronic hepatitis. Gastroenterology. 1993;105:1522–8.
19. Abuaf N, Lunel F, Giral P, et al. Non-organ specific autoantibodies associated with chronic C virus hepatitis. J Hepatol. 1993;18:359–64.
20. Mehta SU, Mishiro S, Segiguchi K, et al. Immune response to GOR, a marker for Non-A, Non-B hepatitis and its correlation with hepatitis C virus infection. J Clin Immunol. 1992;12:178–84.

11
Immune effects of ursodeoxycholic acid

J. NEUBERGER

INTRODUCTION

There is now increasing evidence that therapy with the bile acid, ursodeoxycholic acid (UDCA), plays a significant beneficial role in the treatment of patients with primary biliary cirrhosis (PBC) and may also be of therapeutic benefit in other liver disorders. In patients with PBC, treatment with UDCA is associated with a variable improvement in symptoms (especially of pruritus), a significant improvement in the standard liver tests, a possible retardation of the histological progression, a significant improvement in survival and a reduction in the need for liver replacement. In this chapter, the changes in the immunological variables recorded in patients receiving UDCA and some of the *in-vitro* studies evaluating the mechanisms of these effects will be described.

SEROLOGICAL CHANGES IN PATIENTS RECEIVING UDCA

PBC is characterized by widespread disturbance of the immune system. The two characteristic abnormalities are elevation of serum immunoglobulins (especially IgM) and the antimitochondrial antibody (AMA). Several studies have noted that, in patients receiving UDCA, there is a fall in serum IgM; thus, for example, the Canadian study[1] noted a fall of 18% in serum IgM in treated patients compared with only 0.13% in placebo patients. This change took place during the first three months of therapy and was not associated with changes in either serum IgG or IgA. In contrast, Combes *et al.* found a more modest reduction in serum IgM, that was more marked in those with less-advanced disease and the fall continued over 2 years[2].

Although AMA are virtually diagnostic of PBC, their role in the pathogenesis remains uncertain and no definite evidence of a pathogenetic role has been produced to date. However, therapy with UDCA appears to be associated with alterations in levels of AMA. Yamazaki and colleagues[3] followed 42 patients with PBC for a minimum of 24 months on treatment with UDCA (300–600 mg/day). AMA were quantified by indirect immunofluorescence. Of the 42 patients, AMA became undetectable (titres of 1:10 or less) in 12 (29%); those with lower pretreatment titres of AMA were more likely to become negative. Giner and colleagues[4], in a smaller study, suggested that falls in AMA were more common in the elderly with PBC than in younger patients. The significance of these findings, however, remains unclear. Kisand and colleagues[5] also documented IgG, IgM and IgA antibodies to pyruvate dehydrogenase using ELISA; in PBC patients receiving UDCA, there was a statistically significant fall in the IgA and IgG anti-PDH but no effect on IgM anti-PDH. In contrast, patients receiving placebo or colchicine showed no change in titre of anti-PDH of any isotype.

Other circulating abnormalities are improved in patients with PBC receiving UDCA. Ikeda *et al.*[6] studied the effect of UDCA on circulating lymphocyte subsets in PBC: 15 patients were followed for 1 year and then treated with UDCA 600 mg/day for a further 12 months. In those with PBC, there was a reduction in the proportion of cytotoxic T cells, suppressor/inducer T cells and crp-bearing cells compared with controls. Although no changes in the proportions of these cells were documented over the year on placebo, after 12 months' treatment with UDCA, the proportions of these cells returned to those found in normal individuals. The normalization of the changes in these lymphocyte subsets paralleled an improvement in liver tests. Slightly differing results were reported by Kurktschiev *et al.*[7]: lymphocyte markers were assessed in 22 patients with PBC receiving UDCA: the proportion of $CD4^+$ and $CD8^+$ lymphocytes remained static during the first 20 weeks of therapy while the proportion of $CD26^+$ cells (a marker of IL-2-producing lymphocytes) rose from 9.5% to 21%, reaching values seen in healthy controls after only 8 weeks' therapy. Although levels of soluble IL-2 receptor in serum did not change, *in-vitro* studies of IL-2 production by pokeweed mitogen-stimulated lymphocytes from PBC patients increased from very low levels to normal levels within 12 weeks.

Both peripheral and liver eosinophilia is recognized as a feature of PBC. Yamazaki and colleagues[8] documented a reduction in the circulating peripheral eosinophil count; in 22 patients with PBC, an absolute (>400 cells/μl) and relative (>6%) eosinophilia was found in 32% and 55%, respectively. Serum levels of the major eosinophilic granule proteins were increased at the start of the study, with serum levels of major basic protein (MBP) 963 ± 96 ng/ml and eosinophil-derived neurotoxin (EDN) 50.9 ± 9.2 ng/ml. After 4 weeks treatment with a relatively modest dose of UDCA (300–600 mg/day), the eosinophil count was significantly reduced from 6.2% to 3.0%, and serum MBP fell to 730 ng/ml and EDN to 28.2 ng/ml. Thus, treatment with UDCA is associated not only with a significant fall in serum eosinophilia but with altered function. The mechanisms of these changes and their significance for the liver, however, remain uncertain.

Soluble intercellular adhesion molecule-1 is overexpressed in the liver of patients with PBC, especially on the bile duct cells. The soluble levels of ICAM-1 were assessed in 24 patients before and after treatment with UDCA (10 mg kg^{-1} day^{-1}). There was a statistically significant fall in serum c-ICAM-1 levels of 20%. Some patients were subsequently given additional immunosuppression with corticosteroids and azathioprine, which was associated with a further fall of 25%[9]. Although lymphocyte expression of the activation marker CD25 (interleukin-2 receptor) is increased in patients with PBC, there is no demonstrable effect of UDCA[10].

The extent to which UDCA affects immune cells is variable; thus Calmus and colleagues[11] studied the effect of UDCA on monocyte procoagulant activity, which is a lymphocyte-dependent model of monocyte activation and said to reflect cell-mediated immunity[12]. Although chenodeoxycholic acid had a dose-dependent inhibitory effect on procoagulant activity of endotoxin-stimulated and unstimulated mononuclear cells, no such effect was apparent with UDCA; indeed, the authors concluded that UDCA was devoid of effects on the immune system.

HISTOLOGICAL CHANGES ASSOCIATED WITH UDCA THERAPY IN PBC

Several studies have suggested that histological progression is slowed by treatment with UDCA; however, the slow progression of PBC, the relatively short period of trials and the patchiness of the lesions have made formal assessment less reliable. Treatment with UDCA is associated with a number of histological changes in the liver, both in MHC expression and in cell proliferation. However, Batts *et al.*[13] were unable to demonstrate any changes in histological inflammatory activity in livers of patients with PBC after 2 years' treatment with UDCA, although they did record a weak but statistically significant association between the changes in inflammation and degree of enrichment of UDCA ($r = -0.34$, $p = 0.02$).

Rudi and colleagues[14] used proliferating cell nuclear antigen (PCNA) and Ki-67 to study hepatocyte proliferation in patients with PBC before and after UDCA therapy. Hepatocyte proliferation was higher in PBC liver than in controls and was greater in the earlier stages of the disease. After 3 years treatment with UDCA, the pro-liferation was slightly reduced (for PCNA, from a median of 9.0% to 7.8%, normal <0.5%; and, for Ki-67, from 2.5% to 2.1%, normal <0.5%). Whether these falls are significant clinically is uncertain.

In the normal liver, MHC Class I antigens are expressed by hepatic sinusoidal cells and biliary epithelial cells but not by hepatocytes. In contrast, Class II MHC antigens are expressed by hepatic sinusoidal cells and by dendritic cells. In PBC, there is aberrant expression of both Class I and Class II MHC antigens. Thus, hepatocytes show increased expression of Class I MHC antigens and biliary epithelial cells show increased amounts of both Class I and Class II antigen expression; this increased expression by the biliary epithelial cells is patchy and probably increases with progression of the disease. Calmus *et al.*[15] studied the Class I and II expression of MHC in PBC livers before and after treatment with UDCA. While Class I expression was considerably reduced in those patients treated with UDCA, no effect was noted on MHC Class II antigen expression by biliary epithelial cells. As discussed below, some of these observations may be seen in patients with bile duct ligation, and reflect the consequences of cholestasis and the effect of UDCA on altering the bile acid pool.

The immune consequences of these alterations are uncertain[16]. The major target of the immune response in PBC is the biliary epithelial cells, and Class II MHC antigen expression has been implicated in the pathogenesis of autoimmunity. Reduction in Class I expression by hepatocytes could reduce the ability of the hepatocyte to act as a target for cytotoxic T cells, reduce periportal and lobular hepatocellular necrosis and thus reduce parenchymal damage in PBC. It is more problematic to understand how such alterations in the hepatic expression of MHC lead to less damage to the bile ducts.

IN-VITRO STUDIES WITH UDCA

The studies detailed above indicate clearly that treatment of patients with PBC is associated with improvement in many of the immune abnormalities in patients with PBC, yet these studies do not indicate whether these immune changes are a direct consequence of UDCA on the immune cells or whether UDCA acts indirectly, such as because of the alterations in the bile acid pool. As with all bile acids, there is the potential for *in-vitro* results to be affected by the direct toxicity of bile acids.

UDCA studies on PBLs from normal individuals

The effects of UDCA on human peripheral blood mononuclear cells from normal healthy individuals has been assessed. Thus Lacaille and Paradis[17] examined the effect of UDCA and other bile acids on thymidine incorporation by PBLs stimulated by phytohaemagglutinin (PHA) and by phorbolmyristic acetate (PMA). While no significant inhibition on proliferation was seen at lower concentrations of bile acid (5 μmol/L), at greater concentrations, inhibition was more marked with 15% at 25 μmol/L in the PHA-stimulated system; however, both chenodeoxycholic acid and tauro-UDCA induced more inhibition than UDCA. The inhibitory effect of the bile acids was more marked in the PMA-stimulated system than the PHA system. Pre-incubation of the lymphocytes, prior to stimulation with mitogen, further increased the inhibitory effect – by about 10%. Incubation of the PBLs with bile acids was not associated with any change in the cell-surface expression of antigens, such as IL-2R, transferrin receptor or HLA-DR. However, IL-2 production by PHA-stimulated PBLs was reduced by incubation with UDCA.

These results clearly indicate that bile acids can affect, at pharmacological concentrations, immunomodulatory effects on PBLs, although the effect of UDCA is relatively weak compared with other bile acids. That the same effect was observed when the bile acid was added 24 h after the addition of mitogen implies that the effect of bile acids occurs about the time of or just after DNA synthesis.

When the effect of bile acids on the function of monocytes from normal individuals was studied by Calmus *et al.*[18], they found that there was a dose-dependent inhibitory effect of chenodeoxycholic acid on monocyte production of interleukin-1, interleukin-6 and tumour necrosis factor-α, with 50% inhibitory concentration at 60, 80 and 80 μmol/L, respectively. The effect of UDCA was much less, with 50% inhibitory concentrations for the three cytokines of 100, >200 and >200 μmol/L, respectively. UDCA did not reverse the inhibitory effects of chenodeoxycholic acid on the monocytes.

However, not all workers have been able to reproduce these results. In a recent abstract, Bergamini and colleagues[19] studied the effect of UDCA and other bile acids on cytokine release by isolated human monocytes taken from healthy individuals. In the absence of stimulation, cytokine release was minimal. With LPS stimulation, neither UDCA nor other bile acids had any effect on the stimulated release of either TNFα or IL-6. In contrast, incubation of the cells with dexamethasone had a marked inhibitory effect. Why these results do not confirm those of earlier studies is not clear.

The effect of UDCA on immunoglobulin production by PBMCs was studied by Yoshikawa and colleagues[20] using a plaque assay and stimulation by *Staphylococcus aureus* Cowan I as a stimulant of Ig production. UDCA, at a concentration of 0.01 mmol/L, reduced only IgG production, but, at concentrations of 0.05 mmol/L and above, had a significant effect in reducing production of all three Ig classes. The effect of UDCA was more pronounced than that of tauro-UDCA. These workers also found that incubation of PBMCs from normal individuals with UDCA also suppressed IL-2 and IL-4 production by con A and interferon-γ production induced by poly-I-C, but no effect of UDCA on IL-2 or IL-4 production was observed when the cells were induced by LPS. The authors suggest that UDCA may act, in part, by an effect on T lymphocytes as UDCA will decrease the production of three cytokines (IL-4, IL-2 and IFNγ) that may stimulate Ig production by lymphocytes. Saeki and colleagues have found broadly similar results[21]. Inteferon-γ production by peripheral blood mononuclear cells was studied in controls, PBC patients treated with UDCA and untreated PBC patients. Interferon production by cells from untreated PBC patients was found to be significantly elevated, whereas results in treated PBC patients were similar to those observed in healthy controls. While chenodeoxycholic acid induced interferon production by mononuclear cells from normal individuals in a dose-dependent fashion, this could be reduced by the addition of UDCA. Thus, UDCA may act by inhibiting the effect of other more toxic bile acids. As these and others have reported, the reduction of IL-2 production and the inhibition of IL-1-stimulated thymocyte proliferation by UDCA may point to a more widespread effect of UDCA on the cells of the immune system.

UDCA appears to have an effect also on natural killer cells. Nishigaki *et al.*[22] showed that UDCA treatment significantly increases natural killer cell activity in patients with PBC; they also reported that UDCA increases natural killer cell activity I lymphocytes from normal subjects, whereas other hydrophobic acids reduced NK activity. They suggested that the effect of UDCA was mediated by alteration of the bile acid pool in PBC. They also showed that the secretion of prostaglandin E_2 by lymphocytes from healthy volunteers was reduced.

Although there are no direct data in the liver, Amdt and colleagues[23] have suggested that UDCA attenuates leukocyte–endothelial adhesion. In a rat model of intestinal inflammation induced by indomethacin, these workers found that pretreatment of rats with UDCA (10 mg kg^{-1} day^{-1}) not only had a significant effect on reducing the adherence of adherent and emigrated leukocytes, but was also associated with a significant reduction in both macroscopic and microscopic inflammation.

Effect of UDCA on hepatocytes

As indicated above, livers from patients with PBC have increased HLA expression of MHC antigens, raising the possibility that such aberrant expression may be implicated in antigen expression. Although the antimitochondrial autoantigen is expressed on the membrane of biliary epithelial cells, which are the target of PBC, much research has concentrated on the factors which regulate MHC expression in hepatocytes. It is likely that aberrant MHC expression is due in part to cholestasis: whether this is due to a direct or indirect effect of bile acids (such as mediated by TNF) is uncertain. Calmus *et al.*[24] showed that, in patients with extrahepatic cholestasis, there is increased MHC Class I but not Class II antigen expression. In rat studies, similar results were found and it was noted that neither corticosteroids nor cyclosporine affected HLA expression; neither cholestasis nor immunosuppressive drugs affected the very low expression by hepatocytes of MHC Class II.

The effects *in vitro* of bile acids on hepatocyte HLA expression have been studied using both human and rat hepatocytes. Hillaire *et al.*[25] measured the effect of bile acids on the expression of HLA Class I antigens *in vitro* on isolated human hepatocytes taken from patients without cholestasis. Whereas chenodeoxycholic acid did induce increased expression of HLA Class I antigens, no effect was observed with UDCA. The level of mRNA for Class I was found to parallel the expression of Class I antigens on the membrane; blocking of transcription by actinomycin D inhibited MHC Class I expression whereas incubation with cyclohexamide had no effect. Subsequent experiments suggested that the increased expression of Class I MHC was mediated by the protein kinase system. Incubation of rat hepatocytes with PMA (a PKA activator) and with forskolin (a PKC activator) induced enhanced MHC Class I mRNA as did bile acids. Co-incubation with H7 (a pharmacological inhibitor of both PKC and PKA) inhibited both bile acid and PMA and forskolin-induced mRNA levels. These results suggest that Class I MHC antigen enhancement is induced through the protein kinase system.

Guldutuna and colleagues[26] isolated rat hepatocytes and studied the effect of UDCA on MHC Class I and II expression with and without stimulation with interferon-γ and with differing results. They reported that incubation of the hepatocytes with bile acids had no effect on Class I antigen expression although interferon-induced expression of MHC Class II antigens was significantly reduced by UDCA.

Effect of UDCA on biliary epithelial cells

Gökce and colleagues studied the effect of bile acids on HLA expression in human gall bladder epithelial cells[27]. Gall bladder epithelial cells were isolated by collagenase digestion and grown to confluence. Cells were incubated with a variety of bile acids and the degree of HLA expression determined by staining with FITC-conjugated antibody and analysed by FACs. In untreated gall bladder epithelial cells, there was marked expression of Class I but not Class II MHC. Addition of UDCA (100 and 250 μmol/L) led to a reduction of Class I and II expression, being more marked for Class II (about 25%). After stimulation with IFNγ, UDCA reduced HLA expression by approximately 9%.

We studied the effect of bile acids on the MHC expression of human biliary epithelial cells isolated from normal subjects and from patients with PBC and other chronic liver diseases[28]. Biliary epithelial cells (BECs) were isolated by collagenase digestion and immunomagnetic separation. Phenotypic studies showed that these cells were from the middle-sized portal tracts and not from proliferating bile ductules. Class I and II expression was assessed using fluorescein antibody and the degree of fluorescence measured semiquantitatively. We found that BECs isolated from PBC liver had a higher constitutive expression of both MHC Class I and II than cells isolated from normal liver. *In-vitro* stimulation with both IL-1 and interferon resulted in a significant increase in MHC Class I and Class II expression. Although stimulation with TNFα did result in increased antigen expression, this did not reach statistical significance.

The effect of UDCA was studied in further experiments: biliary epithelial cells were incubated with UDCA, either before or with interferon stimulation. We found that UDCA reduced the intensity of Class I MHC expression when given with but not after interferon. In contrast, UDCA reduced Class II expression at both time points[29].

These results do suggest that UDCA can modulate, *in vitro* at least, membrane MHC expression and may have a direct modulating effect *in vivo*. That no such effect was observed *in vivo* (see above) suggests that this mechanism may not operate *in vivo* or may be too small an effect to be detected.

Mechanism of action of UDCA

UDCA may exert a direct effect on the immune system by a number of mechanisms. Some of the studies discussed above suggest that UDCA has a direct effect *in vitro* on immune cells.

Nitric oxide plays a pivotal role in the regulation of the immune system, not only in non-specific defence mechanisms against pathogens but also in signalling between macrophages and T cells[30]. CD4 lymphocytes may be subdivided into Th1 and Th2, distinguished by the pattern of cytokine secretion: Th1 cells produce IL-2, TNF-β and IFNγ, whereas Th2 produce IL-4, IL-5 and IL-10. The Th1 cells mediate antibody-dependent cell-mediated cytotoxicity and delayed-type hypersensitivity, induce procoagulant activity by monocytes and activate macrophages. In contrast, Th2 cells provide optimal help for B cells and are involved in the expression of vascular adhesion molecules (VCAM-1). Cytokine secretion from one type of Th cells inhibits the other. Acute and local infections with viruses and bacteria are associated with a Th1-type response while chronic infections are associated with a Th2-type response. PBC is associated with a Th1 response although the pattern is not totally clear.

Nitric oxide is implicated in the interaction between Th1 and Th2 cells: Th1 cells, activated by mitogens or antigens, express large amounts of inducible nitric oxide synthetase (iNOS) and produce significant amounts of nitric oxide; this will inhibit Th1 proliferation and production of IL-2. Thus, production of large amounts of nitric oxide will inhibit Th1 expansion and reduce IL-2 production and alter the Th1/Th2 balance. Although there are relatively few studies of the distribution and involvement of nitric oxide in liver disease, its probable importance and role is suggested by, for example, studies in liver allograft rejection. Tox *et al.*[31] showed a different pattern of distribution of immune-reactive inducible nitric oxide synthase in acute and chronic allograft rejection, being distributed variously in hepatocytes, macrophages and inflammatory cells. Control sections showed relatively little nitric oxidase synthase reactivity. Hattori *et al.*[32] studied the effects *in vitro* of UDCA on the synthesis of nitric oxide on J774 macrophages. Although, at the higher concentrations of UDCA used (>250 μmol/L), there was some degree of cytotoxicity observed, at lower concentrations, it was found that UDCA inhibited nitric oxide production in a dose-dependent fashion. It is likely that UDCA acts at the level of nitric oxide synthase as UDCA had no effect on the activity of NOS that was already induced and, while LPS led to a significant reduction in NOS mRNA, this reduction was significantly reduced by UDCA. Similar results were found by Invernizzi and colleagues[33] in a cell line derived from human colonic adenocarcinoma. Cells were incubated with UDCA at the relatively high concentrations of 0.25–1.0 mmol/L before or after stimulation with IFNα or IL-1β. Pretreatment of the cells with UDCA markedly reduced nitric oxidase production in a dose-dependent manner, with nearly 90% reduction at 1.0 mmol/L. Addition of UDCA 6 h after stimulation had no effect.

An alternative or additional mode of action is through interaction with protein kinases. Cellular metabolism is mediated, in part, by a variety of external ligands which exert their effect by binding to specific ligands on the plasma membrane[34]. Most receptors (steroid hormones are the exception, being located in the nucleus) are located on the membrane. Interaction sets in train a signalling cascade involving transducers (G proteins), effector enzymes (adenylate cyclase and phospholipase), second messenger molecules (such as calcium, cyclic AMP, diacylglycerol), primary target kinases (protein kinase A, C, G), intermediate kinases (Raf, MAP kinases) and the final target. The protein kinases were first identified with a role in cell proliferation, but it is now appreciated that their role is far wider, involving, amongst other functions, cell–cell interactions and gene expression. PKC activity is increased not only in many cancers but also in immune diseases, such as asthma and rheumatoid arthritis. It has been demonstrated that PKC activation is involved in MHC expression in hepatocytes (see above) but UDCA does have an effect on some PKC isoenzymes: in a rat model of colon cancer induced by azoxymethane, UDCA administration blocks the induced redistribution of PBC-β2 and PKC-ζ as well as down-regulating PKC-ζ activity[35]. In hamster hepatocytes, while bile acids have no effect directly on cAMP production, UDCA reduces the amount of cAMP formed after stimulation with glucagon[36]; UDCA also induced protein kinase C translocation from cytosol to membrane and stimulated phosphorylation of a protein substrate of 80 kDa, for PKC. Thus bile acids inhibit glucagon-induced cAMP synthesis by uncoupling the glucagon receptor and G(s), mediated by PKC. Whether these observations can be extrapolated to the beneficial effects of UDCA in PBC and whether the effects of UDCA seen in these studies can be extrapolated to immune cells is uncertain, although this effect does not appear to be limited to hepatocytes and may be seen in human umbilical vein endothelial cells and skin fibroblasts[37].

UDCA does have other effects at the genetic level. Weitzel *et al.*[38] examined UDCA activation of the glucocorticoid receptor in isolated rat hepatocytes. In a series of elegant experiments, isolated rat hepatocytes were transfected with a luciferase-reported construct containing the glucocorticoid-responsive element within a mouse tumour promoter. Incubation of these transfected cells with either dexamethasone or UDCA showed only a very weak or no activation of the glucocorticoid receptor. However, when the hepatocytes had been transfected with a glucocorticoid receptor-expressing plasmid, there was a 12-fold increase in luciferase activity after incubation with dexamethasone and a smaller increase when these cells were incubated with UDCA – up to 5-fold with UDCA at concentrations up to 100 μmol/L. Activation of the glucocorticoid receptor results in the release of two 90-kDa heat shock proteins. Thus, in this model, UDCA is able to interact with the glucocorticoid receptor and this may explain some of its immune effects. However, the HSP-70 is reduced in the liver after UDCA therapy[39]. In similar studies, Tanaka and colleagues[40] used cloned hamster ovary cells in which the glucocorticoid receptor was stably integrated. UDCA was found to promote nuclear translocation in a ligand-independent fashion. Transient transfection experiments showed that UDCA marginally increased glucocorticoid-responsive gene expression. Finally, these workers were able to demonstrate that UDCA suppressed IFNγ-mediated induction of MHC Class II expression via the glucocorticoid receptor-mediated pathway.

Thus, while UDCA may have an effect on mRNA and transcriptional activity of genes, this is unlikely to be direct. Kren *et al.*[41] studied the effects of feeding bile acids on mRNA for a wide variety of proteins in hepatocytes. Feeding rats with 1% deoxycholic acid resulted in decreases in mRNA for albumin, the asialoglycoprotein receptor, connexins and various cytochromes, there were increases in mRNA for c-jun, H-ras, fibronectin and some procollagens. Although UDCA had almost no effect on gene expression, it almost completely inhibited the changes associated with deoxycholic acid feeding.

CONCLUSIONS

There is little doubt that UDCA is associated with significant improvement in the serology, biochemistry and progression of primary biliary cirrhosis. Equally, it is clear that, with treatment, there is a normalization of many immune abnormalities, including a reduction in the levels of immunoglobulins and a fall in antimitochondrial antibody titres. Although there is little change in the numbers of CD4 and CD8 cells, there is alteration of some cell types and a variable reduction in the levels of serum markers of immune activation. In the liver, there is a reduction in the hepatocyte expression of MHC Class I antigen but little effect on the bile duct expression of MHC antigens. *In-vitro* studies have shown that UDCA does have a variable effect but some effects observed may arise as a consequence of cytotoxicity. However, UDCA can be shown to induce alterations at the genetic level in a number of situations; the extent to which these are relevant to the beneficial therapeutic effect of UDCA remains uncertain.

References

1. Heathcote EJ, Cauch-Dudek K, Walker V et al. The Canadian multicentre double-blind randomised controlled trial of ursodeoxycholic acid in primary biliary cirrhosis. Hepatology. 1994;19:1149–56.
2. Combes B, Carithers R, Maddrey W et al. Randomised, double-blind, placebo controlled trial of ursodeoxycholic acid in primary biliary cirrhosis. Hepatology. 1995;22:759–66.
3. Yamazaki K, Nakamura A, Abe S, Abe K, Suzuki K, Sato S. Disappearance of antimitochondrial antibody in primary biliary cirrhosis during long-term treatment with ursodeoxycholic acid therapy. Gastroenterology. 1996;110:A1364.

4. Giner R, Gonzalzez O, Terradez J et al. Primary biliary cirrhosis in elderly, long-term treatment with ursodeoxycholic acid (UDCA). Gastroenterology. 1995;108:A1072.
5. Kisand K, Karvonen A, Vuoristo M et al. Ursodeoxycholic acid treatment lowers the serum level of antibodies against pyruvate dehydrogenase and influences their capacity for the enzyme complex in patients with primary biliary cirrhosis. J Mol Med. 1996;74:269–74.
6. Ikeda T, Sato C, Noguchi O et al. Improvement of peripheral blood lymphocyte subsets in primary biliary cirrhosis after ursodeoxycholic acid therapy. J Gastroenterol Hepatol. 1996;11:366–72.
7. Kurktschiev D, Subat S, Adler D, Schentke K. Immunomodulating effect of ursodeoxycholic acid therapy in patients with primary biliary cirrhosis. J Hepatol. 1993;18:373–7.
8. Yamazaki K, Nakamura A, Suzuki K, Sato S, Kita H, Gleich G. Serum eosinophil granule-associated protein concentration in primary biliary cirrhosis. Hepatology. 1995;22:122A.
9. Lim AG, Wolfhagen F, Verma A et al. Soluble intercellular adhesion molecule 1 in primary biliary cirrhosis: effect of ursodeoxycholic acid and immunosuppressive therapy. Hepatology. 1995;22: 124A.
10. Lim A, Jazrawi R, Petroni M, Pereira S, Maxwell J, Northfield T. Interleukin-2 receptor expression in primary biliary cirrhosis. Gut. 1994;35 Suppl. 4:1010.
11. Calmus Y, Podevin P, Robert A, Poupon R. Differential effects of chenodeoxycholic and ursodeoxycholic acids on the expression of procoagulant activity by human monocytes. J Hepatol. 1994;20: 446–72.
12. Halloran P, Aprile M, Haddad G, Robinette M. Procoagulant activity in renal transplant recipients. Transplantation. 1985;39:374–81.
13. Batts K, Jorgensen R, Dickson E, Lindor K. Effects of ursodeoxycholic acid on hepatic inflammation and histological stage in patients with primary biliary cirrhosis. Am J Gastroenterol. 1996; 91:2314–17.
14. Rudi J, Waldherr R, Raedsch R, Kommerell B. Hepatocyte proliferation in primary biliary cirrhosis as assessed by proliferating cell nuclear antigen and Ki-67 labelling. J Hepatol. 1995;22:43–9.
15. Calmus Y, Gane P, Rouger P, Poupon R. Hepatic expression of class I and class II major histocompatibility complex molecules in primary biliary cirrhosis: effect of ursodeoxycholic acid. Hepatology. 1990;11:12–15.
16. Lindor K. What is the role of major histocompatibility complex expression in cholestasis? Gastroenterology. 1992;102:1429–30.
17. Lacaille F, Paradis K. The immunosuppressive effect of ursodeoxycholic acid: a comparative in vitro study on human peripheral blood mononuclear cells. Hepatology. 1993;18:165–72.
18. Calmus Y, Guechot J, Podevin P, Bonnefis M, Giboudeau J, Poupon R. Differential effects of chenodeoxycholic and ursodeoxycholic acids on interleukin 1, interleukin 6 and tumour necrosis factor-α production by monocytes. Hepatology. 1992;16:719–23.
19. Bergamini A, Dini L, Falasca L et al. Bile salts do not influence cytokine production by human monocytes and murine Kupffer cells. Gastroenterology. 1996;110:A1151.
20. Yoshikawa M, Tsuji T, Matsumura K et al. Immunomodulatory effects of ursodeoxycholic acid on immune responses. Hepatology. 1992;16:358–364.
21. Saeki R, Ogino H, Kaneko S, Unoura M, Kobayashi K. Effects of chenodeoxycholic and ursodeoxycholic acids on interferon-gamma production by peripheral blood mononuclear cells from patients with primary biliary cirrhosis. J Gastroenterol. 1995;30:739–44.
22. Nishigaki Y, Ohnshi H, Moriwaki H, Muto Y. Ursodeoxycholic acid corrects defective natural killer activity by inhibiting prostaglandin E(2) production in primary biliary cirrhosis. Dig Dis Sci. 1996;41:1487–93.
23. Amdt H, Palitzsch K-D, Kullman F, Gross V, Grune S, Scholmerich J. Ursodeoxycholic acid attenuates leukocyte–endothelial cell adhesion in indomethacin-induced intestinal inflammation in the rat. Gastroenterology. 1995;108:A774.
24. Calmus Y, Arvieux C, Gane P et al. Cholestasis induces major histocompatibility complex class I in hepatocytes. Gastroenterology. 1992;102:1371–7.
25. Hillaire S, Boucher E, Calmus Y et al. Effects of bile acids and cholestasis on major histocompatibility complex class I in human and rat hepatocytes. Gastroenterology. 1994;107:781–8.
26. Guldutuna S, Bhatti, Gokce Y, Leuchner U. Effect of bile salts on HLA class I and class II antigen expression on isolated rat hepatocytes. J Hepatol. 1996;25:167S.
27. Gokce Y, Gultutuna S, Hottenrott U, Leuschner U. The in vitro effect of bile salts on HLA antigens of human gallbladder epithelial antigens (GBECs). J Hepatol. 1996;25:167S.
28. Ayres R, Neuberger J, Shaw J, Joplin R, Adams D. Intercellular adhesion molecule-1 and MHC

antigens on human intra-hepatic bile duct cells – effect of pro-inflammatory cytokines. Gut. 1993;34:1245–9.
29. Neuberger J, Joplin R. MHC expression in liver and the effect of bile acids. In: Berg PA, Leuschner U, Eds. Bile Acids and Immunology. Dordrecht: Kluwer Academic Publishers; 1995:131–9.
30. Barnes P, Liew F. Nitric oxide and asthmatic inflammation. Immunol Today. 1995;16:128–30.
31. Tox U, Burkhard M, Goester T, Arnold J, Stremmel W, Thielmann L. Distribution of inducible nitric oxide synthase in liver tissue after liver transplantation. Hepatology. 1995;22:361A.
32. Hattori Y, Murakami Y, Hattori S, Kuroda H, Kasai K, Shimoda S. Ursodeoxycholic acid inhibits the induction of nitric oxide synthase. Eur J Pharmacol. 1996;300:147–50.
33. Invernizzi P, Salman A, Setchell K. Ursodeoxycholic acid inhibits induction of the human intestinal epithelial nitric oxide synthase. Hepatology. 1995;22:361A.
34. Lord J, Pongracz J. Protein kinase C: a family of isoenzymes with distinct roles in pathogenesis. Clin Mol Pathol. 1995;48:M57–M64.
35. Wali R, Bissonnette M, Khare S. Chemoprotective ursodeoxycholic acid but not chemopromotional cholic acid, prevents the activation of PKC-β2 and PKC-ζ in the azoxymethane model of colon cancer. Gastroenterology. 1995;108:A550.
36. Bouscarel B, Gettys T, Fromm H, Dubner H. Ursodeoxycholic acid inhibits glucagon-induced cAMP formation in hamster hepatocytes – a role for PKC. Am J Physiol Gastro Liver Physiol. 1995;31:G300–10.
37. Bouscarel B, Ceryak S, Gettys T, Fromm H, Noonan F. Alterations of cAMP-mediated hormonal responsiveness by bile acids in cells of non-hepatic origin. Am J Physiol Gastro Liver Physiol. 1995;31:G908–16.
38. Weitzel C, Gosl D, Scholmerich J, Holstege A. Ursodeoxycholic acid induced activation of glucocorticoid receptor in primary rat hepatocytes. J Hepatol. 1996;25:133S.
39. Sakisaka S, Koga H, Kuboyama S, Uchimura Y, Sata M, Tanikawa T. Reduced expression of heat shock protein in the primary biliary cirrhosis liver after ursodeoxycholic acid treatment. Hepatology. 1995;22:483A.
40. Tanaka H, Makino Y, Miura T et al. Ligand-independent activation of the glucocorticoid receptor by ursodeoxycholic acid – repression of IFN-gamma induced MHC class II expression via a glucocorticoid receptor dependent pathway. J Immunol. 1996;156:1601–8.
41. Kren B, Rodrigues C, Setchell K, Steer C. Posttranscriptional regulation of messenger-RNA levels in rat liver associated with deoxycholic acid feeding. Am J Physiol Gastro Liver Physiol. 1995;32:G961–73.

12
Immunosuppressive therapy of autoimmune hepatitis

I. G. McFARLANE

INTRODUCTION

In many autoimmune diseases, only a proportion of patients respond to immunosuppressive drugs, and often only partially. In contrast, almost all patients with autoimmune hepatitis respond quite rapidly and can be maintained in remission for long periods on low doses of these drugs. Indeed, the response is such a striking feature of the disease that, at the World Congresses of Gastroenterology in Los Angeles in 1994, an international panel[1] was prompted to include it as part of the following definition of autoimmune hepatitis (AIH):

> *'An unresolving, predominantly periportal hepatitis, usually with hypergammaglobulinaemia and tissue autoantibodies, which is responsive to immunosuppressive therapy in most cases.'*

Notwithstanding this satisfactory response, however, it is important to remember that AIH is a potentially serious life-threatening condition. Before the advent of effective therapy, it was known to progress rapidly to cirrhosis and some reports indicated that up to 50% of patients died within two years and up to 80% within five years of diagnosis[2–5]. Since the introduction of effective therapy around 1970, the 5-year mortality has fallen to less than 10% and, in fact, a recent study at the Mayo Clinic has indicated that the life-expectancy in carefully managed patients (with or without cirrhosis) is not significantly different from that in an age- and sex-matched normal population[6]. There is also an impression that treatment slows progression to cirrhosis but there are not yet any definitive data to support this.

The controlled clinical trials conducted in the late 1960s and early 1970s at the Mayo Clinic and at the Royal Free and King's College Hospitals in London[4,5,7], demonstrated very clearly that the disease can be effectively controlled with corticosteroids and that, if azathioprine is used in combination, the dose of corticosteroids needed to maintain control can be significantly reduced. This became, and still is, the standard therapy.

A number of other drugs (D-penicillamine, cyclophosphamide, cyclosporin, tacrolimus, ursodeoxycholic acid) have been tried over the years but, of these, only D-penicillamine has been subjected to controlled clinical trials[8,9]. These trials showed that D-penicillamine is as effective as corticosteroids for maintaining remission once this has been induced by corticosteroids but it is associated with a number of adverse side-effects and offers no advantages over corticosteroids. There are only isolated reports of the efficacy of the other drugs mentioned above but it is worthwhile to bear all of these in mind because they might be useful in the few cases that prove difficult to control on standard therapy. Ursodeoxycholic acid (UDCA) is particularly interesting in view of recent reports that it may have some immunosuppressive effects[10]. A Japanese group[11] has reported marked symptomatic and biochemical improvement in four patients treated with UDCA and we have found this also in three patients that we treated recently. However, there are not yet any data to indicate that UDCA therapy leads to histological improvement.

Treatment with prednisolone and azathioprine was originally developed on an entirely empirical basis, but there is now much evidence to indicate that there is a sound mechanistic basis for the efficacy of these drugs in AIH. Data from several animal models and from *in-vitro* studies using T cells cloned from patients' liver biopsies suggest that liver damage in AIH may involve direct T-cell cytotoxic reactions against hepatocytes[12–16]. However, it is doubtful whether results from such animal models and other artificial systems can be extrapolated to the human situation. Certainly, these findings do not mirror observations in patients. In the late 1970s and early 1980s, studies by several groups around the world failed to demonstrate T-cell cytotoxicity against autologous hepatocytes in patients with AIH. All of these groups, however, found that they could easily demonstrate so-called antibody-dependent cytotoxic (ADCC) reactions against appropriate target cells *in vitro* in the patients (for reviews see References 17 and 18). Support for ADCC as an important mechanism of liver damage *in vivo* comes also from the observation that hepatocytes obtained from liver biopsies from AIH patients are coated with antibodies and that this is associated with ADCC reactions[19].

The ADCC mechanism initially involves recognition by helper T cells of an autoantigen on the surface of the target cell. The T cells become activated and can instruct B cells to produce autoantibodies against the antigen. This process is thought to be part of the normal mechanism of immune surveillance. It is under the control of regulatory/inhibitor ('suppressor') T cells and production of autoantibodies is normally 'switched off'. Patients with AIH, however, appear to have a defect in this control mechanism[20]. As a consequence, large quantities of autoantibodies against liver antigens are produced and some of these can bind to the surfaces of hepatocytes. Killer (K) cells, a non-T lymphocyte subpopulation with the ability to recognize antibodies when they are bound to antigens, can then damage the hepatocytes.

Corticosteroids exert their effects on the immune system mainly through the T cells, and act at several points during the process of T-cell recognition of antigen, antigen processing and activation of T cells[21–24]. They do not appear to act directly on B cells to any significant extent, but the net effect of their complex actions at the T cell level is to switch off production of immunoglobulins, including autoantibodies, by the B cells. Azathioprine, in contrast, seems to have little or no action against T or B cells and exerts its effects mainly by depleting the numbers of natural killer (NK) and K cells in the circulation[25–27]. In combination, therefore, these two drugs effectively control the two main components of the ADCC reaction. However, whereas the action of corticosteroids is very rapid, the effects of azathioprine develop much more slowly and it takes several months for the numbers of circulating K cells to be reduced to very low levels.

TREATMENT STRATEGIES

Because treatment with corticosteroids and azathioprine is usually so effective in AIH, and is so easy to administer, many physicians have developed their own preferred treatment regimens. These differ according to the precise dosages of the drugs, intervals between administration and duration of therapy, but they can be grouped under three main headings:

- Lifetime immunosuppression,
- Symptomatic treatment,
- Intermittent therapy.

There is a view that, since more than 80% of patients relapse sooner or later when all treatment is stopped[28,29], most patients will require some form of immunosuppressive therapy for very long periods – perhaps for life. An alternative view is that, once the disease is well controlled, patients need to be treated only when they are symptomatic or have biochemical or histological evidence of active disease, and that treatment should be withdrawn and reinstituted as and when necessary if the patient relapses. The third approach, intermittent therapy, relates to the practice of giving the drugs either in alternating doses or the same dose on alternate days, or in pulses of high doses at intervals of one or two weeks. In two separate studies, the Mayo Clinic has shown that this approach does not effectively control the disease[30,31], which has been our experience also. The poor efficacy of intermittent therapy probably relates to the quite short (only a few hours) biological half-lives of these drugs and, consequently, only partial control is achieved by such regimens.

Undoubtedly, severe symptomatic AIH requires prompt immunosuppressive treatment. Less certain is the question of whether patients with milder disease should be treated[32]. This is still the subject of a debate[33,34] which seems to hinge on: (a) whether there is indeed a distinct subgroup of patients with so-called 'mild' AIH whose disease will not progress in the absence of therapy, and (b) how to identify these cases. The difficulty in identifying such cases relates to the well-known fluctuating nature of the condition, which may enter long periods of treatment-induced or spontaneous remission only to flare up (often acutely) later, and the unreliability of symptoms and serum biochemical liver tests as indices of disease severity[35,36]. Most leading authorities today would agree that it is probably safer to treat all cases of AIH[34].

Perhaps the main reason for the existence of so many different approaches to therapy relates to concerns about the well-recognized adverse side-effects of these drugs, particularly when used in the long term (Table 1). Consequently, there is considerable pressure on the clinician to reduce or stop treatment as soon as possible. However, too rapid reduction or withdrawal of treatment frequently results

Table 1. Potential complications of corticosteroid and azathioprine therapy

Corticosteroids	*Azathioprine*
Minor	Minor
Cushingoid facies	Malaise
Rashes (acneiform)	Nausea/vomiting
Weight gain	Rashes
Serious	Serious
Cataracts	Hepatotoxicity
Diabetes	Carcinogenicity
Hypertension	Teratogenicity
Osteoporosis	Myelosuppression
Psychoses	

in early relapses. Relapses can be quite sudden and severe and fatalities have occurred when treatment has not been re-started promptly. Therefore, very careful monitoring is required during and after treatment withdrawal.

INDUCTION OF REMISSION

In recent years, several of the major centres where significant numbers of AIH patients are seen have independently evolved similar treatment strategies that almost approach a consensus. The salient points are:

(1) Aggressive initial treatment to control the disease as quickly as possible,

(2) Careful reduction of corticosteroids once remission is established,

(3) Maintenance of remission for a long period on low-dose corticosteroids with azathioprine before attempting to withdraw treatment, and

(4) Very gradual withdrawal of treatment thereafter.

In these centres, treatment is usually initiated with prednisone or prednisolone at a dose of approximately 0.5 mg kg^{-1} day^{-1} (20–40 mg/day). It may sometimes be necessary to use higher doses, especially in younger patients with severe disease, but this increases the risk of development of the more serious side-effects (see below). The use of lower doses (< 15 mg/day) initially, with subsequent incremental increases if the response is not satisfactory, does not control the disease adequately and may prolong the period during which there is ongoing liver damage. Azathioprine should be introduced early, either from the outset or within two or three weeks after starting steroids because, as noted above, it takes 3–6 months for this drug to become fully effective. Also, early introduction of azathioprine facilitates planning of subsequent management if the drug is not tolerated.

When the serum aminotransferase (AST or ALT) and globulin (or IgG) levels have become normal (usually within 1–2 months), the prednisolone dose is reduced stepwise to 15 mg/day (with azathioprine at 1 mg kg^{-1} day^{-1}). Patients should then be maintained on this dose for a further 1–3 months (to ensure that these parameters remain normal) before reducing the steroids (at the rate of not greater than 2.5 mg/day monthly) to 10 mg/day. If after three months the AST/ALT and globulins (or IgG) are still normal, consideration may be given to further reducing the steroids to a final maintenance level of between 5 and 10 mg/day. In practice, it is advisable to use the highest dose within this range that the patient will tolerate, and they should then be maintained on this dose with azathioprine (1 $mg\,kg^{-1}\,day^{-1}$) for at least one year (and preferably two years) unless complications develop (see below).

LONG-TERM MANAGEMENT

Opinion varies about how to proceed after the patient has been in clinical and biochemical remission for one or two years on the above maintenance regimen. Most authorities agree, however, that histological remission should be confirmed (if possible) before any major changes in therapy are contemplated. If complete remission is assured, many physicians prefer then to very slowly withdraw all treatment and re-introduce therapy as above when patients relapse. In our experience, the large majority of patients will relapse sooner or later and we take the view that each relapse increases the risk of progression to cirrhosis or exacerbation of existing cirrhosis. We therefore prefer to continue immunosuppressive therapy for as long as possible. Thus, when complete remission has been sustained for two years, we double the dose of azathioprine[37] to approximately 2 $mg\,kg^{-1}\,day^{-1}$. After one or two months, if this higher dose is tolerated, the prednisolone is gradually withdrawn at the rate of 2.5 mg/day monthly and the patient is maintained thereafter on 2 $mg\,kg^{-1}\,day^{-1}$ azathioprine alone. In a 10-year follow-up of 72 of our patients treated in this way, 83% sustained remission on the higher dose of azathioprine alone. This contrasts with our previous experience that 93% relapse when all treatment is withdrawn[37]. Unfortunately, not all patients can be maintained on azathioprine alone. For reasons that we believe may be related to genetic variations in the metabolism of this drug (see below), about 20% of our patients continue to require low doses of corticosteroids to sustain remission. After one or two years on the higher dose of azathioprine, in many cases, it is possible to reduce the dose back to the conventional level of 1 $mg\,kg^{-1}\,day^{-1}$ but about 25% relapse on this lower dose and careful monitoring is therefore required.

COMPLICATIONS AND THEIR MANAGEMENT

The main complications that arise with corticosteroids and azathioprine relate to the adverse side-effects of these drugs (Table 1). In our experience with the above regimen, about 50% of patients develop the minor side-effects of steroid therapy. Only about 10% develop more serious complications, mainly non-insulin-dependent diabetes and hypertension (exacerbated by the weight gain), but it is not always certain that these are directly related to the treatment. The cosmetic changes usually resolve when steroids are withdrawn, and the accompanying weight loss is also often associated with improvement of hypertension[38].

Approximately 10% of our patients experience minor side-effects (Table 1) when azathioprine is first introduced at the conventional dose, necessitating discontinuation of the drug. However, in about half of these cases, the symptoms do recur when the drug is reintroduced again at a low dose (25 mg/day) after a few months, and usually they subsequently tolerate the higher doses.

Up to 50% of patients maintained on azathioprine alone develop a non-inflammatory arthritis after stopping steroids[37]. It affects the finger, elbow and knee joints, and may last for up to a few months. The arthralgia seems to be related to withdrawal of the steroids rather than to the azathioprine and, in most cases, it can be relieved by mild analgesia (paracetamol) but occasionally non-steroidal anti-inflammatory drugs are required.

Azathioprine is said to be hepatotoxic, and it has been implicated in the development of nodular regenerative hyperplasia[39]. There is also evidence to suggest that the drug might be carcinogenic[40,41]. Most of this evidence comes from studies in transplant recipients, and it is not strongly supported by evidence from studies of the use of azathioprine in other situations, such as in the treatment of rheumatoid arthritis[42]. Furthermore, azathioprine has now been used for treating AIH for more than 25 years, and there have not yet been any reports of major problems relating to these two adverse effects. Certainly our data suggest that, if there is a risk, it seems to be small[37]. There is also a theoretical possibility that the drug might be teratogenic, although most authorities feel that the risk to a fetus associated with a relapse of AIH during pregnancy is much higher than that associated with azathioprine therapy[43]. Nonetheless, our current practice with women receiving azathioprine who plan to become pregnant is to re-introduce or increase the dose of steroids, and then withdraw the azathioprine. In any event, if azathioprine has to be discontinued for any reason, it is important to remember that the drug is given for its 'steroid-sparing' effects and a compensatory increase (or re-introduction) of the steroids will be required to maintain remission.

Myelosuppression is the only serious side-effect of azathioprine therapy that we have seen in any significant number of patients. This develops in about 5% of our cases during the first year of treatment with azathioprine at 1 $mg\,kg^{-1}\,day^{-1}$. A further 5% tolerate this dose but develop myelosuppression on the higher dose. However, it is important to distinguish true myelosuppression from leucopenia and thrombocytopenia due to hypersplenism, which is common in these patients. This distinction can be made relatively easily by regularly monitoring the full blood count (FBC). In cytopenia due to hypersplenism, the low white cell and platelet counts remain stable whereas in true myelosuppression there is a progressive decrease in cell counts over a relatively short period of time. Lymphopenia is also very common in these patients, but it seems to be a feature of the disease rather than of the treatment because we have found no significant difference in lymphocyte counts between patients taking azathioprine and those receiving prednisolone alone[37].

The reason why myelosuppression develops in only a small proportion of patients at the doses used in AIH relates to common genetic polymorphisms in one of the enzymes involved in metabolism of the drug. Azathioprine is normally first converted non-enzymatically in the blood to 6-mercaptopurine and then, by hypoxanthine–guanine phosphoribosyl transferase (HGPRT), to 6-thioguanine nucleotides (6-TGNs), which are the active metabolites that exert the immunosuppressive and cytotoxic effects of the drug[44]. An alternative pathway, involving the action of the enzyme thiopurine methyltransferase (TPMT), converts azathioprine and 6-mercaptopurine to inactive metabolites. However, about 11% of the population are heterozygous and about 1 in 300 are homozygous for an allele that encodes an inactive form of TPMT. Such individuals have very low

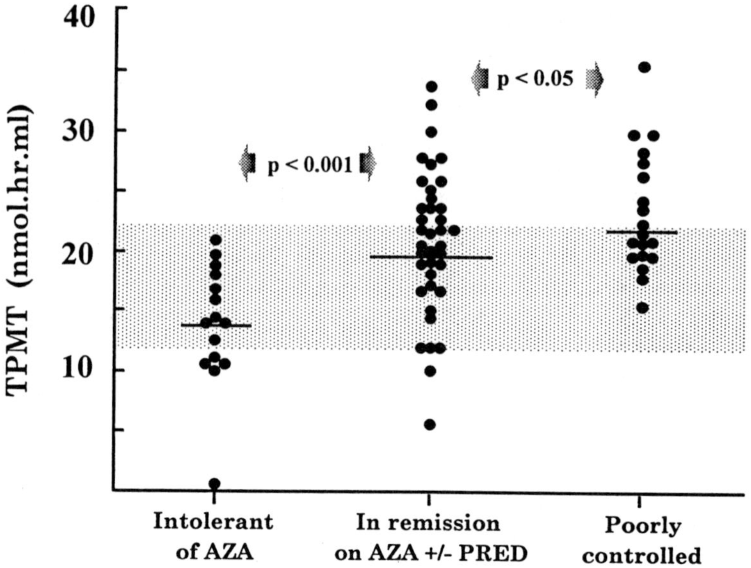

Figure 1. Thiopurine methyl transferase (TPMT) activities in erythrocytes of patients with autoimmune hepatitis. Patients who sustained remission on azathioprine (either at 2 mg kg^{-1} day^{-1} alone or at conventional doses in combination with prednisolone at 5–10 mg/day) had significantly higher TPMT levels than those who were intolerant of the drug (development of myelosuppression or other side-effects). In the latter group, note one patient with undetectable levels of TPMT who developed aplastic anaemia within three weeks of treatment with 50 mg/day azathioprine. The third group comprised patients who tolerated azathioprine but relapsed whenever prednisolone was reduced below 10 mg/day and were difficult to maintain in remission. These patients had significantly higher TPMT activities than either of the other two groups

TPMT activities and, consequently, most of the drug is converted to the highly toxic 6-TGNs. Conversely, some individuals have very high levels of TPMT activity and rapidly detoxify most of the administered azathioprine.

Recent data from our Institute suggest that the genetic polymorphisms determining TPMT activity may account for the differences in responses to azathioprine between individual patients with AIH. Patients who were intolerant of the drug (i.e. they developed either myelosuppression or the minor side-effects) were found to have significantly lower TPMT levels than those who tolerated the drug and were successfully maintained on either the higher dose of azathioprine alone or at the conventional dose in combination with low-dose (5–10 mg/day) prednisolone (Figure 1). One patient in the former group had undetectable levels of TPMT, and is presumably a homozygote for the allele encoding inactive TPMT. This patient developed aplastic anaemia within three weeks of receiving 50 mg/day of azathioprine. A third group of patients tolerated azathioprine but their disease was difficult to control because they relapsed whenever their prednisolone dose was reduced below 10 mg/day. These patients were found to have significantly higher TPMT levels than either of the other two groups, which suggests that they may be detoxifying the drug too rapidly for it to be effective at the doses used. If a rapid test for TPMT activity can be developed, as suggested by Ben Ari *et al.*[45], it would be useful to screen AIH patients to identify (a) those with low activities who are likely to develop azathioprine-induced myelosuppression or other side-effects, and (b) those with high TPMT activities who might need higher doses of the drug.

CONCLUDING REMARKS

Because the standard immunosuppressive therapy for AIH is now well established, it is tempting to regard management of this disease as relatively straightforward. This is not the case. AIH is quite heterogeneous with respect to its presentation, subsequent course and response to therapy. All patients need to be carefully monitored in the long term (probably for the rest of their lives) and each needs to be treated as an individual. For example, a modest rise in serum aminotransferase or IgG levels may be of little consequence in one patient but highly significant and herald relapse in another. The rewards of careful management can be seen in the resulting significant reduction in morbidity and mortality, as noted in the report from the Mayo Clinic mentioned above[6].

References

1. International Working Party Report. Terminology of chronic hepatitis. Am J Gastroenterol. 1995; 90:181–9.
2. Wilcox RG, Isselbacher KJ. Chronic liver disease in young people. Clinical features and course of thirty-three patients. Am J Med. 1961;30:185–95.
3. Mistilis SP, Skyring AP, Blackburn CRB. Natural history of active chronic hepatitis. Aust Ann Med. 1968;17:214–23.
4. Soloway RD, Summerskill WHJ, Baggenstoss AH et al. Clinical, biochemical and histological remission of severe chronic active liver disease: a controlled study of treatments and early prognosis. Gastroenterology. 1972;63:820–33.
5. Cook GC, Mulligan R, Sherlock S. Controlled prospective trial of corticosteroid therapy in chronic active hepatitis. Q J Med. 1971;40:159–85.
6. Roberts SK, Therneau TM, Czaja AJ. Prognosis of histologic cirrhosis in type 1 autoimmune hepatitis. Gastroenterology. 1996;110:848–57.
7. Murray-Lyon IM, Stern RB, Williams R. Controlled trial of prednisolone and azathioprine in active chronic hepatitis. Lancet. 1973;1:735–7.
8. Stern RB, Wilkinson SP, Howorth PJN, Williams R. Controlled trial of synthetic D-penicillamine and prednisone in maintenance therapy for active chronic hepatitis. Gut. 1977;18:19–22.
9. McClements BM, Callender ME. D-Penicillamine therapy in patients with HBsAg-negative chronic active hepatitis and major prednisolone-induced adverse effects. J Hepatol. 1990;11:322–5.
10. Reichen J. Analysis of experimental data on the concept of interactions between bile salts and immunological effector reactions. In: Berg PA, Leuschner U, Eds. Falk Symposium No. 86: Bile Acids and Immunology. Dordrecht: Kluwer; 1996:281–9.
11. Mima S, Sekiya C, Kanagawa H, Uchida T. Ursodeoxycholic acid (UDCA) therapy for auto-immune hepatitis. Int Hepatol Commun. 1994;2:207–12.
12. Mori T, Mori Y, Yoshida H et al. Cell-mediated cytotoxicity of sensitized spleen cells against target liver cells – in vivo and in vitro study with a mouse model of experimental autoimmune hepatitis. Hepatology. 1985;5:770–7.
13. Ogawa M, Mori Y, Mori T et al. Adoptive transfer of experimental autoimmune hepatitis in mice – cellular interaction between donor and recipient mice. Clin Exp Immunol. 1988;73:276–82.
14. Kohda H, Sekiya C, Kanai M et al. Flow cytometric and functional analysis of mononuclear cells infiltrating the liver in experimental autoimmune hepatitis. Clin Exp Immunol. 1990;82:473–8.
15. Tiegs G, Hentschel J, Wendel A. A T cell-dependent experimental liver injury in mice inducible by concanavalin A. J Clin Invest. 1992;90:196–203.

16. Wen L, Peakman M, Mowat AP et al. $\gamma\delta$+ T cell clones from liver biopsies of children with autoimmune chronic active hepatitis (ACAH) and primary sclerosing cholangitis (APSC) are cytotoxic to human liver target cells. J Hepatol. 1991;13:S80 (abstract).
17. McFarlane IG. Editorial review: Autoimmunity in liver disease. Clin Sci. 1984;67:569–78.
18. Vento S, Eddleston ALWF. Immunological aspects of chronic active hepatitis. Clin Exp Immunol. 1987;68:225–32.
19. Vergani D, Mieli-Vergani G, Mondelli M et al. Immunoglobulin on the surface of isolated hepatocytes is associated with antibody-dependent cell-mediated cytotoxicity and liver damage. Liver. 1987;7:307–15.
20. Vento S, O'Brien CJ, McFarlane IG et al. T-cell inducers of suppressor lymphocytes control liver-directed autoreactivity. Lancet. 1987;1:886–7.
21. Arya SK, Wong-Staal F, Gallo RC. Dexamethasone-mediated inhibition of human T cell growth factor and gamma interferon messenger RNA. J Immunol. 1984;133:273–6.
22. Lew W, Oppenheim JJ, Matsushima K. Analysis of the suppression of IL-1 alpha and IL-1 beta production in human peripheral blood mononuclear adherent cells by glucocorticoid hormone. J Immunol. 1988;140:1895–902.
23. Boumpas DT, Anatassiou ED, Older SA et al. Dexamethasone inhibits human interleukin-2 but not interleukin-2 receptor gene expression in vitro at the level of nuclear transcription. J Clin Invest. 1991;87:1739–47.
24. Sierra-Honigmann MR, Murphy PA. T cell receptor independent immunosuppression induced by dexamethasone in murine T helper cells. J Clin Invest. 1992;89:556–60.
25. Shih WWH, Ellison GW, Myers LW et al. Locus of selective depression of human natural killer cells by azathioprine. Clin Immunol Immunopathol. 1982;23:672–81.
26. Prince HE, Ettenger RB, Dorey FJ et al. Azathioprine suppression of natural killer activity and antibody-dependent cellular cytotoxicity in renal transplant recipients. J Clin Immunol. 1984; 4:312–18.
27. Pedersen BK, Beyer JM, Rasmussen A et al. Azathioprine as single drug in the treatment of rheumatoid arthritis induces complete suppression of natural killer cell activity. Acta Pathol Microbiol Immunol Scand [C]. 1984;92:221–5.
28. Hegarty JE, Nouri-Aria KT, Portmann B et al. Relapse following treatment withdrawal in patients with autoimmune chronic active hepatitis. Hepatology. 1983;3:685–9.
29. Czaja AJ, Beaver SJ, Shiels MT. Sustained remission after corticosteroid therapy of severe hepatitis B surface antigen-negative chronic active hepatitis. Gastroenterology. 1987;92:215–19.
30. Summerskill WHJ, Korman MG, Ammon HV et al. Prednisone for chronic liver disease: dose titration, standard dose, and combination with azathioprine. Gut. 1975;16:876–83.
31. Czaja AJ, Wang KK, Shiels MT, Katzman JA. Oral pulse prednisone therapy after relapse of severe autoimmune chronic active hepatitis. A prospective randomized treatment trial evaluating clinical, biochemical and lymphocyte subset responses. J Hepatol. 1993;17:180–6.
32. Koretz RL, Lewin KJ, Higgins J et al. Chronic active hepatitis: who meets treatment criteria? Dig Dis Sci. 1980;25:695–9.
33. Yarze JC. Autoimmune hepatitis. N Engl J Med. 1996;334:923 (letter).
34. Meyer zum Buschenfelde KH, Lohse AW. Autoimmune hepatitis. N Engl J Med. 1996;334: 923–4 (letter).
35. McFarlane IG. Clinical spectrum and heterogeneity of autoimmune hepatitis: an overview. In: Meyer zum Buschenfelde KH, Hoofnagle JH, Manns M, Eds. Falk Symposium 70 – Immunology and Liver. Dordrecht: Kluwer; 1993:179–92.
36. Hay JE, Czaja AJ, Rakela J, Ludwig J. The nature of unexplained chronic aminotransferase elevations of a mild to moderate degree in asymptomatic patients. Hepatology. 1989;9:193–7.
37. Johnson PJ, McFarlane IG, Williams R. Azathioprine for long-term maintenance of remission in autoimmune hepatitis. N Engl J Med. 1995;333:958–63.
38. Stellon AJ, Keating JJ, Johnson PJ et al. Maintenance of remission in autoimmune chronic active hepatitis with azathioprine after corticosteroid withdrawal. Hepatology. 1988;8:781–4.
39. Gane E, Portmann B, Saxena R et al. Nodular regenerative hyperplasia of the liver graft after liver transplantation. Hepatology. 1994;20:88–94.
40. Viteri A, Vernace SJ, Schaffner F. Extrahepatic malignancy in chronic liver disease: report of six cases. Gastroenterology. 1976;71:1075–8.
41. Wang KK, Czaja AJ, Beaver SJ, Go VL. Extrahepatic malignancy following long-term immunosuppressive therapy of severe hepatitis B surface antigen-negative chronic active hepatitis. Hepatology. 1989;10:39–43.

42. Silman AJ, Petrie J, Hazleman B, Evans SJ. Lymphoproliferative cancer and other malignancy in patients with rheumatoid arthritis treated with azathioprine: a 20 year follow up study. Ann Rheum Dis. 1988;47:988–92.
43. Witter FR, King TM. Drugs and the management of chronic diseases in the pregnant patient. In: Stern L, Ed. Drug Use in Pregnancy. Balgowlah, Australia: AIDS Health Science Press; 1984: 190–211.
44. Johnson PJ. Immunosuppressive drug mechanisms. In: McFarlane IG, Williams R, Eds. The Molecular Basis of Autoimmune Hepatitis. Austin, Texas: RG Landes; 1996:177–91.
45. Ben Ari Z, Mehta A, Lennard L, Burroughs AK. Azathioprine-induced myelosuppression due to thiopurine methyltransferase deficiency in a patient with autoimmune hepatitis. J Hepatol. 1995; 23:351–4.

Index